AF556166

NEEM
THE VILLAGE PHARMACY

Neeraj Pratap Singh
M.Sc.(Horticulture), MBA
5/839, Viram Khand, Gomti Nagar
Lucknow (UP) India

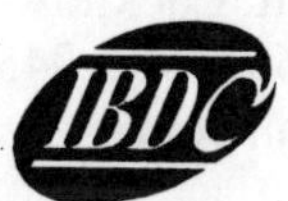

International Book Distributing Co., India
(Publishing Division)

Published by

International Book Distributing Co.

(Publishing Division)
Khushnuma Complex Basement
7, Meerabai Marg (Behind Jawahar Bhawan)
Lucknow 226 001 U.P. (INDIA)
Tel. : 91-522-2209542, 2209543, 2209544, 2209545
Fax : 0522-4045308
E-Mail : ibdco@airtelmail.in

First Edition 2009

ISBN 81- 8189-161-9

Composed & Designed at :
Panacea Computers
3rd Floor, Agrawal Sabha Bhawan
Subhash Mohal, Sadar Cantt. Lucknow-226 002
Phone : 0522-2483312, 9335927082, 9452295008
E-mail : prasgupt@rediffmail.com

Printed at:
Salasar Imaging Systems
C-7/5, Lawrence Road Industrial Area
Delhi - 110 035
Tel. : 011-27185653, 9810064311

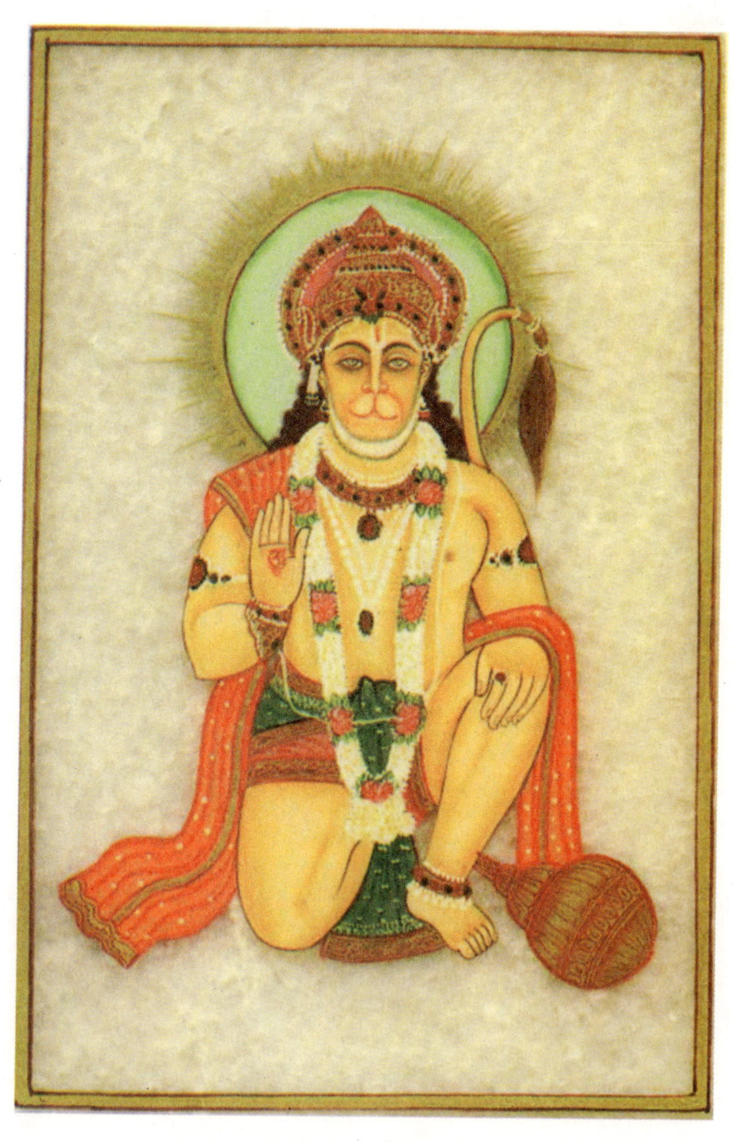

तेरा तुझको अर्पण

Preface

For thousands of years humans have sought to fortify their health and cure various ills with herbal remedies. Throughout this time, the search for a true panacea or cure-all has been undertaken by virtually every civilization. While hundreds of substances have been tried and tested, few have withstood modern scientific scrutiny. Perhaps no other botanical meets the true definition of a panacea than *Neem*, a tropical evergreen native to India.

When the indentured immigrants came to the Caribbean to toil the land, they brought with them their knowledge of plants. Today, many of the plants used for their medicinal and culinary values by the indentured East Indians are still finding their place in everyday use. One of these is the wonder plant, *Neem*.

Every part of this fascinating plant has been used to treat hundreds of different maladies from ancient to modern times. While it is still revered in India for its superior healing properties, recent investigation has dramatically increased worldwide interest in *Neem* and the many products now manufactured with this almost miraculous herb.

In India the *Neem* tree has been revered as the 'village pharmacy", where it has served the people faithfully for centuries. Every part of this sacred tree is used in some form on a daily basis - the twigs as a toothbrush, the oil for soap, and the leaves for medicine. The diversity of *Neem's* uses is staggering. It is commonly used in the manufacture of natural medicines, health and beauty preparations, culinary seasonings and natural insect repellents.

The Ayurvedic literature is replete with references to *Neem's* genuine effectiveness for a myriad of ailments. In "The Yoga of Herbs", Vasant Lad and David Frawley say, "Neem is one of the most powerful blood-purifiers and detoxifiers in Ayurvedic usage. It cools the fever and clears the toxins involved in most inflammatory skin diseases." They describe the actions of *Neem* as: antipyretic (fever reducing), alterative (produces gradual beneficial change in body), anthelmintic (dispels parasites), antiseptic (destroys bacteria), and bitter tonic (strengthens the organism).

Michael Tierra, in his herbal classic, "The Way of Herbs," further adds the properties of astringent (firms tissues and organs) and anti-inflammatory to the previous description. He says, "An extract of the leaves and bark has powerful antibacterial and antiviral activity. It is also taken internally to eliminate worms". The leaf extracts and oil from the seed kernel has also been used for centuries by Indians to maintain beautiful and healthy skin.

We may be familiar with *Neem* as a culinary spice, or you may have purchased *Neem*-based toothpastes. This is only the beginning of the *Neem* story. Consumers can soon expect to find a complete selection of products containing *Neem* such as cremes, lotions, tinctures, extracts, and capsules.

In addition to its numerous uses as a healing agent, *Neem* has been receiving much attention for the ecological benefits it provides. For centuries Indians have been mixing *Neem* leaves with stored grains to prevent insect infestation. But *Neem* is not simply a natural alternative to pesticides; increasingly it is being used to reverse desertification and to reduce erosion and deforestation, making it an important weapon in the fight against global warming. *Neem's* many practical applications make it of enormous interest to anyone concerned about health and ecology.

Ongoing scientific research is validating what Ayurvedic practitioners have known for centuries; *Neem* is a dynamic and useful plant which can solve dozens of problems, while enhancing overall well being.

The book **Neem –'The 'Village Pharmacy'** gives maximum synopsis of the world's most amazing plant; neem. This comprehensive review on *Neem* is an excellent collation of many therapeutic and ecological uses of neem. It is a definitive resource that will be of interest to everyone involved in the subjects like horticulture, landscaping, botany, phytochemical, ecology & environment, agronomy, entomology and biopesticide.

Neeraj Pratap Singh

Contents

Chapter 1

The Tree

Botanical Description

Classification

Common Name: NEEM (also Margosa)

Kingdom :	Plantae
Division	Magnoliophyta
Class:	Magnoliopsida
Order :	Sapindales
Family :	Meliaceae
Genus :	Azadirachta
Species :	A. indica
Scientific Name :	Azadirachta indica L. (syn. *Antelaea azadirachta, Melia azadirachta, Melia indica*).

The latinized name of Neem - Azadirachta indica - is derived from the Persian:

Azad = Free, dirakht = Tree, i - Hind = of Indian Origin which literally means: 'The Free Tree of India'.

NAMES OF NEEM IN INDIA AND AROUND THE WORLD

Hindi – Neem, Nimb

Urdu: nim, neem

Sindi: nimmi

Bengali - Nim, Nimgachh

Konkani - Beva-rooku

Marathi - Kadunimb

Gujarati - Leemdo

Tamil - Vembu, Vempu, Veppan

Punjabi – Nimb, Neem

Malayalam - Veppu, Aryaveppu, Aruveppu, Kaippan, Veppu, Vepa

Simhalee - Nimu

Oriya - Nimo

Telegu - Vepa

Kannada - Bevinmar, Kahibevu

Sanskrit: nimba, nimbou, arishtha (reliever of sickness)

Kiswahili: Mwarubaini(Muarobaini)

English - Margosa, Neem, Indian Lilac

French: azadira d'Inde, margousier, azidarac, azadira

Sri Lanka: kohomba

German - Indischer Zadrach, Niembaum

Persian - Azade Darakhte Hindi(Free Tree of India), Nib

Arabic - Azad Darkhtu Hind

Burmese - Tamabin, Kamakha,Tamar, Tamarkha

Malay - Dawoon Nambu, Veppa

Latin - Azadirachta indica A. Juss or Melia azadirachta Linn

Farsi - Azad darkht 1 hindi (Free tree of India)

Singapore - Kohumba, nimba

Indonesia - Mindi

Nigeria - Don goyaro

Spanish – Margosa, Nim

Nepal - Nim

Portuguese – Margosa(Goa), Nimbo

Use

Although largely uncultivated, Neem is the source of a wide variety of products including adhesives, beauty aids, fertilizers, herbs, lumber, pesticides, and numerous pharmaceuticals. These products are variously derived from the bark, leaves and seeds. In the dry season, the leaves are used as cattle feed. Cultivation of neem for fire wood, proposed since the 19th century, has been limited. Cultivation for oil extracts is largely unexplored. Extracts of Neem, often called "Nature's drugstore", have been used in medicine for over 2,500 years and perhaps much longer. Neem oil components, especially azadirachtin, have potential for use as pesticides because they inhibit molting, feeding and reproduction in phytophagous insects. Neem produces a small fruit, about 3/4 in long, having a yellowish sweet pulp surrounding a small brown seed. The pulp is believed to be edible.

Plant:

The Neem trees are attractive broad-leaved ever greens that grow up to a height of 12 to 25 m tall and 2.5 m in girth. Their spreading branches form rounded crowns as much as 20 m across. They remain in leaf except during extreme drought, when the leaves may fall off. The short, usually straight trunk has a moderately thick, strongly furrowed bark.

Its use as a slow growing shade tree in landscaping and as a house plant is increasingly popular. The leaves are dark green and slender with resin secreting glands on young leaves near the shoot apex. The bark on young branches is green, but grey to grey black on the main trunks. Extra floral nectaries are present at the base of leaf petioles and on the adaxial side of leaflets. Neem thrives in the tropics with an extended dry season, is drought tolerant, and loses its leaves following moisture or cold stress. The taproot (at least in young specimens) may be as much as twice the height of the tree. The roots penetrate the soil deeply, at least where the site permits, and, particularly when injured, they produce suckers. This suckering tends to be especially prolific in dry localities. It requires well drained soils, but tolerates poor soils and extreme heat. The tree may live for more than two centuries.

Inflorescence:

Blossoms begin to develop on trees that are 3 - 5 years old and the tree is reproductively mature after ten years. The flowers are bisexual, pentamerous, regular, small, whitish pink and borne on axillary cymose panicles. Flower buds open in the afternoon and evening producing a strong scent at night. The 0.2 in (5 mm) long protandrous flowers have a sweet jasmine-like fragrance and produce ample quantities of nectar. Their scent attracts many bees. Neem honey is popular, and reportedly contains no trace of azadirachtin- a neem extract used in bio-insecticides.The capitate tri-lobed sticky stigma stands above 3 - 5 bi-ovulate carpels, and at the same level of the ten anthers which are united into a single tube. Each flower matures only a single seed. Like other Meliaceae, neem flowers from January through April with fruit ripening in June through August. A Second minor flowering period may occur from July to October.

Fruit

The edible fruit is an ovoid drupe with a thin mucilaginous sweet pulp up to 2 cm long. The yellow or greenish fruit darkens and becomes wrinkled at maturity and comprises a sweet pulp enclosing a seed. The seed is composed of a shell and a kernel (sometimes two or three kernels), each about half of the seeds weight. It is the kernel that is used most in pest control. (The leaves also contain pesticidal ingredients, but as a rule they are much less effective than those of the seed.).The number of fruit/ seeds per tree is highly variable. Embryo abortion is common. A Neem tree normally begins bearing fruit after 3-5 years, becomes fully productive in 10 years, and from then on can produce up to 50 kg of fruits annually.

Pollination Requirements:

Bisexual and male flowers occur on the same tree. Floral anatomy and the absence of self incompatibility facilitates self pollination via the wind. However, bees are required to effect cross pollination which ensures optimal seed/fruit set and may limit embryo abortion. Neem flowers are fragrant and highly attractive to bees. They are a good nectar source and a minor source of pollen for bees. The size of the pollen grain of *A. indica* (ca 55-65 microns in diameter) is within the size range for bee pollination (Nair, 1965). The role of the extra floral nectaries, if any, in the pollination ecology of neem appears unknown.

Pollinators:

Bees observed visiting the anemophilous neem flowers and effecting self- and cross pollination include *Apis florea, A. cerana, Trigona* spp. and *Ceratina* spp. Existing knowledge suggests that Meliaceous flowers are largely insect pollinated. Although moths normally pollinate several species, members of this family of plants are important sources of pollen and nectar for honey bees. Bees are listed as the major visitors of the flowers of related species, *Swietenia macrophylla* and *Cedrela odorata.*

Pollination Recommendations and Practices:

The cultivation of neem on a large scale for its numerous products has been recommended, especially in dry areas. For this, basic knowledge of the pollination strategies of neem will be required. Pollinator species should be conserved and encouraged to maximize seed set. Clearly, profitable cultivation of neem requires more study of its pollination ecology.

In India, neem trees are a major source of honey bee. Planting of neem is recommended to increase honey production. Neem honey is composed primarily of water, fructose and glucose (22.88%), sucrose (7.46%), ash (0.06%), free acid (20.8 meg/kg). The honey is light amber in color, and its viscosity is low. The taste is good although slightly bitter. Azadirachtin was not detected in neem flowers or green fruit up to 40 days after anthesis.

Chemical analyses for neem pollen are unavailable. However, neem pollen offers intriguing possibilities since all other components of the neem tree have been shown to possess useful properties. Pollen gathered by honey bees from many other plant sources is collected and sold by beekeepers, in various regions of the world, because of its nutritional and pharmaceutical value. Studies should be conducted to determine whether neem pollen is unique in this regard.

OTHER SPECIES OF NEEM

There are two other known distinct species of neem. These are *Azadirachta siamensis* (Syn. *A. azadirachta* var. *siamensis*) and *Azadirachta excelsa*. There are also different ecotypes of each species and crosses between species. For the most part the compounds found in each species of neem tree are the same, though the relative percentages of each compound may vary. However, there are compounds found in each that are unique to the individual species. Further research probably can better define these differences.

A. siamensis

In Thailand, the seeds and young leaves of this species, called "sweet" neem, are used as additions to many foods as spices. The *A. siamensis* compounds are similar to those of the Indian neem but the leaves, which are about twice as large as *A. indica*, are less bitter. The seeds are also considerably larger and the kernels are an emerald green rather than white. The characteristic garlic-like smell is still there and so is the very bitter taste. However, *A. siamensis* has a spicy, hot tinge that supplements the taste of the seed.

The medicinal uses of *A. siamensis* in Thailand are similar to those of *A. indica* in India. Much of the Indian tradition of medicine was carried to Thailand and the rest of south-east Asia by merchants and emigrants over the thousands of years that these ancient cultures have been trading with each other. Neem did not attain the religious significance that it did in India and was not a pervasive influence on the daily life of the Thai people. However, it was recognized for the qualities of healing and good health that neem is known for everywhere.

A. excelsa

There is one other recognized species of neem that grows in remote areas of Malaysia and the Philippine islands called *Azadirachta excelsa*. This species grows upto 160 feet tall deep in the mostly inaccessible rainforests. The tree is protected by the government from logging and the distribution of the seeds is strictly controlled. Due to its rarity and location in remote areas, only scientific or conservation use is permitted and few seeds are allowed out of the country. Because of its scarcity this species of neem, like *A. siamensis*, is not used extensively for commercial products. It is used in some indigenous medicines for such problems as stomach ulcers, skin problems, malaria and as a general tonic against illness. As in Thailand, some of the Indian medical tradition was transferred to these areas by travellers over the centuries. Neem became a part of the combined medical culture of the peoples of these countries.

Though the three species of neem trees differ in appearance, the usefulness of the medicinal compounds in each species was recognized and used by healers throughout south-east Asia. As researchers in these countries begin understanding the true possibilities of these trees, greater emphasis is being placed on protecting the available varieties. They are also promoting the establishment of plantations of neem trees to be able to supply the growing demand for the commercial products that can be obtained from them.

Distribution

Neem is a member of the Mahogany family (Meliaceae) which includes a large array of tropical trees and shrubs native to both the Old and New World.

Neem is thought to have originated in Assam and Burma (where it is common throughout the central dry zone and the Siwalik hills). However, the exact origin is uncertain: some say neem is native to the whole Indian subcontinent; others attribute it to dry forest areas throughout all of South and South east Asia,, i.e. India, Pakistan, Bangladesh, Sri Lanka, Burma, Thailand, Malaysia and Indonesia. In addition neem is found in several other countries spread over continents. Neem now has become a global tree.

It is in India that the tree is most widely used. It is grown from the southern tip of Kerala to the Himalayan hills, in tropical to subtropical regions, in semiarid to wet tropical regions, and from sea level to about 700 m elevation.

Neem was introduced to Africa earlier this century. It was brought from India. Now it is planted extensively in the tropical regions of Africa, particularly in the regions along the Sahara's southern fringe, where it has become an important provider of both fuel and lumber. Although widely naturalized, it has nowhere become a pest. Indeed, it seems rather well "domesticated": it appears to thrive in villages and towns.

In recent times neem has been introduced into Saudi Arabia, Yemen, China (Hainan Island), and Philippines. Small plantings of neem are also found in USA (South Florida and Hawaii), Brazil and Australia. This presence is, however, scattered and exploratory.

Indentured labourers from India carried neem with them as a part of the India heritage to many countries to which they migrate such as in Fiji, Mauritius, the Caribbean, Middle East and many countries of Central and South America. In some cases it was probably introduced by indentured labourers, who remembered its value from their days of living in India's villages. In other cases it has been introduced by foresters. In the continental United States, small plantings are prospering in southern Florida, and exploratory plots have been established in southern California and Arizona.

Climate

The neem has adapted to a wide range of climates. The tree is said to grow "almost anywhere" in the lowland tropics. Neem tree needs little water and plenty of sunlight. It generally performs best in areas with annual rainfalls of 400-1,200 mm. However, it has been introduced successfully even in areas where the rainfall is as low as 200 - 250 mm. It thrives under the hottest conditions, where maximum shade temperature may soar past 50°C, but it will not withstand freezing or extended cold up to 0° C. It does well at elevations from sea level to perhaps 1,500m near the equator.

In northern climates it may be grown in pots with the care and appearance of the more-common Ficus tree. Neem makes an ideal indoor plant because it grows well with a minimum of maintenance. For optimum growth, neem should be placed near a sunny window during the winter and moved outside during summer months. However, they will survive indoors even if they don't receive any natural light at all. They also should be grown in a pot as large as possible or their growth will be stunted to remain proportionate in size with their root system.

Soil

The neem grows on almost all types of soils including clayey, saline and alkaline soils. It is renowned for good growth on dry, infertile sites. It does well on black cotton soil and deep, well-drained soil with good sub-soil water. It performs better than most trees where soils are hard calcareous or clay pan, sterile, stony, and shallow, or on some acid soils. Indeed, it is said that the fallen neem leaves, which are slightly alkaline (pH 8.2), are good for neutralizing acidity, improving fertility and water-holding capacity in the soil. On the other hand, neem cannot stand "wet feet," and quickly dies if the site becomes waterlogged. Whether grown indoors or out, neem trees must have well-drained soil.

Propagation

The tree is easily propagated-both sexually and vegetatively. It can be planted using seeds, seedlings, saplings, root suckers or tissue culture. However, it is normally grown from seed, either planted directly on the site or transplanted as seedlings from a nursery.

The seeds are fairly easy to prepare. The fruit drops from the trees by itself; the pulp, when wet, can be removed by rubbing against a coarse surface; and (after washing with water) the clean, white seeds are obtained. In certain nations-Togo and Senegal, for example people leave the cleaning to the fruit bats and birds, who feed on the sweet pulp and then spit out the seeds under the trees.

It is reputed that neem seeds are not viable for long. It is generally considered that after 2-6 months in storage they will no longer germinate. However, some recent observations of seeds that had been stored in France indicated that seeds without endocarp had an acceptable germinative capacity (42 per cent) after more than 5 years.

Fertilization

They are relatively heavy feeders, responding to organic fertilizers such as fish emulsion, bone meal and kelp with lush new growth. If leaves begin to turn yellow, the tree has been given too much fertilizer or water. Although neem trees are evergreen, they often lose their leaves in very dry periods or after a hard frost. Neem trees will quickly revive with regular watering or the onset of warm summer days.

Growth

Neem often grows rapidly. The neem grows slowly during the first year of planting. Young neem plants cannot tolerate intensive shade, frost or excessive cold. It can be cut for timber after just 5-7 years and becomes fully productive in 10 years.

Neem can take considerable abuse. For example, it easily withstands pollarding (repeated lopping at heights above about 1.5 m) and its topped trunk resprouts vigorously. It also freely coppices (repeated lopping at near-ground level). Re-growth from both pollarding and coppicing can be exceptionally fast because it is being served by a root system large enough to feed a full-grown tree.

Weeds

Weeds seldom affect growth. Except in the case of very young plants, neem can dominate almost all competitors. In fact, the trees themselves may become "weeds." They spread widely under favourable site conditions, since the seeds are distributed by birds, bats, and baboons. For some reason, natural regeneration under old trees is often abundant. But for that, in virtually every place it grows neem is considered a boon, not a ban. People almost always like to see more neems coming up.

Yield

Maximum yields reported from northern Nigeria (Samaru) amounted to 169m3 of fuel wood per hectare after a rotation of 8 years. Yields in Ghana were recorded between 108 and 137m3 per hectare in the same time. A mature tree produces 30- 50 kg. fruit every year.

Insects

By and large, most neem trees are reputed to be remarkably pest free; however, in Nigeria 14 insect species and 1 parasitic plant have been recorded as pests. Few of the attacks were serious, and the trees almost invariably recovered, although their growth and branching may have been affected.

However, in recent years a more serious threat has emerged. In some parts of Africa (mainly in the Lake Chad Basin), a scale insect (*Aonidiella orientalis*) has become a serious pest. This and other scale insects sometimes infest neem trees in central and south India. They feed on sap, and although they do little harm to mature trees, they may kill young ones. Now that one type has been detected in Africa, the impact could be severe.

Other insect pests include the following:

- The scale insect *Pinnaspis strachani* (very common in Asia, Africa and Latin America)
- Leaf-cutting ants *Acromyrmex* sp. (common defoliators of young neem trees in Central and South America)
- The tortricid moth *Adoxophyes aurata* (attacks leaves in Asia including Papua New Guinea)
- The bug *Helopeltis theivora* (considered a serious neem pest in southern India)
- The pyralid moth *Hypsipyla* sp. (attacks neem shoots in Australia)

Even though neem timber is renowned for termite resistance, termites sometimes damage, or even kill, the living trees. They usually attack only sickly specimens, however.

Diseases

Despite the fact that the leaves contain fungicidal and antibacterial ingredients, certain microbes may attack different parts of the tree, including the following:

- Roots (root rot, *Ganoderma lucidum*, for instance)
- Stems and twigs (the blight *Corticium salmonicolor*, for example)
- Leaves (a leaf spot, *Cercospora subsessilis*; powdery mildew, *Oidium* sp., and the bacterial blight *Pseudomonas azadirachtae*)
- Seedlings (several blights, rots, and wilts-including Sclerotium, Rhizoctonia, and Fusarium)

A canker disease that discolours the wood and seems to coincide with a sudden absorption of water after long droughts has also been observed.

Nutrient Deficiencies

Lack of zinc or potassium drastically reduces growth. Trees affected by zinc deficiency show chlorosis of the leaf tips and leaf margins, their shoots exude much resin, and their older leaves fall off. Those with potassium deficiency show leaf tip and marginal chlorosis and die back (necrosis).

Other Problems

Fire kills neem seedlings outright. However, mature trees almost always regrow, especially if the dead parts are quickly cut away.

High winds are a potential problem. Large trees frequently snap off during hurricanes, cyclones, or typhoons. Neem is therefore a poor candidate for planting in areas prone to such violent storms.

Seedlings regenerating beneath stands of neem are sensitive to sudden exposure to intense sunlight. Thus, a clear-felling neem tree normally produces a massive seedling kill, especially if the seedlings are small.

In some localities rats and porcupines kill young trees by gnawing the bark around the base. Even when not causing any physical damage, rodents can be pests: wherever they are numerous, the fruits may disappear before the farmer can harvest them.

Neem, with its intensely bitter foliage, is not a preferred browse, but if nothing else is available goats and camels will eat it. In fact, in Asia goats and camels have been known to browse young neem trees so severely in times of scarcity that the plants died. In Africa neem is generally ignored by livestock (which makes the tree easy to establish even within villages and courtyards). The reason that livestock treat neem differently in Asia and Africa is unknown at present. It may be differences in the tree specimens, or in the animals' preferences or past experiences.

Chapter 2

Establishment

Neem is usually easy to establish. It grows best on deep, well drained sandy soils. However, it often fails on silty or micaceous loams and silty clays, in depressions with slow drainage, and in soils with high or seasonally fluctuating water tables.

In their first months after transplanting from a nursery, neem seedlings greatly benefit from tillage, weeding, irrigation, and one or two fertilizations.

Young plants develop fairly rapidly, at least after the first season. As a rule their girth increases 2-3 cm a year, although even faster growth is often attained.

Neem needs open sunlight for best performance, but seedlings vigorously push their way up through thorny scrub and even crop plants. The seedlings begin by emphasizing root growth. Only when roots are well established does the overhead growth become rapid. In harsh environments and on poor soils, this early emphasis on establishing extensive roots endows the tree with exceptional ability to survive adversity.

Although neem can be raised in nurseries and transplanted as seedlings, direct sowing on the site is sometimes easier and more successful. Seeds should be taken from thoroughly ripe fruits picked directly off the trees. They should be sown as quickly as possible.

ASIA

Neem has been planted in many parts of Asia: Bangladesh, Burma, Cambodia, India, Indonesia, Iran, Malaysia, Nepal, Pakistan, Sri Lanka, Thailand, and Vietnam. It has recently been introduced into Saudi Arabia, the northern plains of Yemen, and China (Hainan Island).

India

In India, neem grows wild in dry forests and is also cultivated in all but the highest, coldest parts of the country. It thrives best in the drier zones of the northwest, and a large number of trees are found in the state of Uttar Pradesh. It is commonly planted as a roadside tree to form shady avenues. Visitors to New Delhi cannot fail to admire the stately neems adorning the avenues, spreading from both sides a thick green canopy that shields people from the fierce sun.

Burma

Although Burma is one of the main countries where neem is native, not much about its neem trees has been recorded. Nonetheless, in recent years a German aid project has helped Burmese scientists develop a neem-seed pesticide. This one-step, formulated, methanolic extract is produced by a pilot factory in Mandalay. The product has become popular among local farmers, who use it for controlling vegetable and peanut pests. The factory also produces neem oil and sells it locally for manufacturing soap and candles.

Indonesia

Java has an enormous array of different types of neem trees. Some growing on a small commercial plantation have recently been found to have seeds that are extraordinarily effective against insects due to their high content of active compounds.

Pakistan

Neem is fairly widespread in the country south of Lahore. In many cities giant neem trees, more than 100 years old and more than 30 m tall, grace many roads.

Phillipines

Neem was introduced to the Philippines only in 1978, by scientists working at the International Rice Research Institute (IRRI). By 1990, however, IRRI had distributed more that 120,000 seedlings and the tree was growing on at least eight islands. Wide-scale plantings for fuel-wood and potential pesticide production had also been undertaken by private and governmental agencies. Owing to numerous typhoons, neem is unsuited to the northern and central regions, but in the south it grows well.

Saudi Arabia

Introduced into the country more than 40 years ago, the tree has acclimated remarkably well to the hot and arid conditions. It is probably more common than date palm or any other tree as an avenue tree and can be seen in Jeddah and other cities.

In the plains where the Prophet Muhammad is said to have delivered his farewell sermon some 1,400 years ago, a city of thousands of tents springs up each year to accommodate the pilgrims. In the area, one of the hottest on earth, there is little relief from the intense heat-but relief is on the way. What is probably the world's largest neem plantation, about 50,000 trees, has recently been planted. The project is designed to provide shade to the 2 million Muslim pilgrims who camp there annually for the hajj.

Thailand

Thailand has many "Indian" neem trees (*Azadirachta indica*) as well as its own species, *Azadirachta siamensis,* which also might have promise. It is fast growing. At Ratchaburi, on and rock outcroppings, 200,000 specimens averaged 11 m tall only 6 years after planting. They were also heavily laden with fruits.

Africa

Indian immigrants introduced neem to Mauritius and may also have taken it to continental Africa. It is now widely cultivated in Mauritania, Senegal, The Gambia, Guinea, Ivory Coast, Ghana, Burkina Faso, Mali, Benin, Niger, Nigeria, Togo, Cameroon, Chad, Ethiopia, Sudan, Somalia, Kenya, Tanzania, and Mozambique. In each case, it is found particularly in the drier, low-lying areas.

Senegal

Because of tree planting programs of the Forestry Department and of the local people, Senegal probably has more neems than any other African country. The tree dominates towns and villages all over the country. It is used for shade and for firewood, and it has very beneficial ecological consequences, including the saving of many indigenous trees that would, in its absence, have been felled for fuel.

Ghana

Neem has been growing on the plains near Ghana's capital, Accra, since the 1920s. The trees have naturalized, and their spread has been boosted by birds and bats that feed on the fruits and spit out the seeds while sitting in the branches. Neem is now scattered all over the area.

With their vigorous growth, the trees have become Ghana's major source of firewood. Alongside many highways and byways, it is common to see stacks of neem wood awaiting trucking to the cities.

In Accra and other centers, neem is now a common street tree and backyard shade tree. It is normally pollarded (topped) annually and the resulting branch wood hawked for fuel or building poles.

How Neem Reached Africa

To people in West Africa these days, neem seems like an established part of the countryside. The general feeling is that it has been there since time immemorial. However, this tree is actually a recent addition to the African scene.

It was Brigadier-General Sir Frederick G. Guggisberg who brought neem to Ghana, for example. He was governor (of what was then known as the Gold Coast) from 1919 to 1927, and he introduced seeds or seedlings from India sometime during that period. The first were planted in the Northern Territories. Today, as a result, neem is found throughout Ghana and the Sahelian region.

The Governor's efforts have given rise to at least two local names for neem. In Ghana, the tree is normally called "king," which is the local title for Governor. In Mali, the vernacular name in the Dyula language is "goo-gay," a corruption of "Guggisberg."

Neem was first introduced to Nigeria in 1928 (probably from Ghana), where it was successfully established in the Bornu province. Several thousand seedlings from the first plantation were replanted in Sokoto, Katsina, and Kano provinces in the 1930s. Neem was also successfully established by sowing fresh seed directly into the shelter of indigenous vegetation and local food crops. There are now considerable plantations for firewood and construction materials throughout those areas of northern Nigeria.

Neem also seems to be an entrenched part of the scene in the Sudan. There, it is valued mainly as a street and amenity tree and is commonly seen at railway stations and beside mosques. Here again, however, neem is a new arrival, historically speaking. The first ones apparently were planted at Shambat in 1916. Probably, they were brought directly from India by a diligent colonial forester who appreciated their value for producing shade, fuel, wood, and oil for lamps.

Just how Senegal got its first neem is uncertain, but in the 1950s Senegalese agronomist Djibril Sene went to India to gather neem seeds. Many, if not most, of the neems now seen throughout the country result from his far-sighted efforts.

Niger

At the beginning of the nineteenth century, the Majjia Valley in central Niger was heavily wooded. But it is located in the southern Sahel, an area with highly variable and low rainfall (400-600 mm a year). The growing population with a relentless appetite for fuelwood, fodder, and construction materials-left it bare. By the drought years of the early 1970s, wind erosion was blowing away nearly 20 tons of topsoil per hectare per year. In the rainy season, wind-blown sediment would smother farmers' seedlings, forcing them to reseed their fields over and over.

In 1975, the American relief agency CARE began planting neem windbreaks. By 1987, some 560 km of double rows of neem were established and more than 3,000 hectares of cropland protected. The trees cut wind velocity near the ground by 45-80 per cent, resulting in less erosion and more soil moisture. Crop yields jumped 15 per cent or more, even after accounting for the land taken up by the lines of trees.

Moreover, the obvious beneficial effect of the windbreaks-particularly as a source of cash from the sale of wood- has encouraged some farmers to start their own nurseries. Currently, more than 100 private nurseries are being tended. The long-term success of the project seems to be assured by the spread of the woodlots and nurseries into private control.

Nigeria

Neem is common, especially in towns and villages, in the northern regions. Sometimes it is planted in large numbers along roadsides along the road between Maiduguri and Lake Chad, for instance.

Mali

Neem is part of the scene along the Niger. Many of the trees are pollarded (at about 2 m height) to provide forage to cattle and goats. Many are also pruned into unusual shapes by camels.

Sudan

Sudan was one of the first African countries to get neem. Today, the trees are widespread along the Blue and White Niles, in irrigation schemes, and in towns and villages.

THE AMERICAS

Apparently, it was immigrants from India who introduced neem to several Caribbean nations. The tree is now grown as a medicinal plant in Suriname, Guyana, Trinidad and Tobago, Barbados, Jamaica, and elsewhere. More recent neem plantings are also found in St. Lucia, Antigua, Dominican Republic, Mexico, Belize, Guatemala, Honduras, Nicaragua, Bolivia, Ecuador, and Brazil. In most of these nations, however, the plantings are small, scattered, and exploratory. Only in Haiti, the Dominican Republic, and Nicaragua have large numbers of neem trees been planted so far.

Haiti

In the last decade or so, neem has been widely planted in Haiti. In fact, this tree is now one of the leading species for reforesting this much-denuded land. For example, one project funded by USAID has planted 200,000 neem trees as part of a road beautification program using seed imported from Africa in the late 1970s. Later, neem became a popular species for planting. The trees have grown so well that today neem seed is becoming a Haitian export. Approximately 40 tons were processed for azadirachtin by an American company in 1990. Since then, other companies have also sought to buy Haiti's neem seed.

United States

Because the tree is a tropical species, it probably cannot be grown economically in the continental United States beyond South Florida. In South Florida, however, there are four mature neem trees (two in Miami and two in Fort Myers) and 50 smaller ones (in Homestead). There are also eight trees in the futuristic Biosphere 2.

Of course, the tree can thrive in Hawaii and other locations in the American tropics. Researchers have already begun planting it in Puerto Rico and the Virgin Islands, for example. A specimen planted at the East-West Center in Honolulu, Hawaii, in 1984 was nearly 10 m tall and fruiting heavily in 1991. And in 1989 the Hawaii State Senate passed a resolution supporting research and development of this "wonder tree."

THE PACIFIC

Nineteenth century immigrants carried the tree from India to Fiji, and it has since spread to other islands in the South Pacific, even to Easter Island, which is hardly known as a place for trees. In Papua New Guinea neem was introduced at the beginning of the 1980s, mainly in the Port Moresby area.

Chapter 3

History

Neem - the legendary medicinal tree of India has grown with the human settlement all over the country and has been an integral part of the Indian way of life for centuries. The history of the neem tree is inextricably linked to the history of the Indian civilization.

The healing properties of neem are spoken about in the Vedas, the world's oldest books, and for almost 5,000 years, millions of Indian people have used all parts of this sacred tree as medicinals - the seeds, leaves, flowers, fruits, oil, roots and bark.

The first indication that neem was being used as a medicinal treatment was about 4,500 years ago. This was the high point of the Indian Harappa culture, one of the great civilizations of the ancient world. Excavations at Harappa and Mohenjo-Daro in North-Western and Western India that date from that period found several therapeutic compounds, including neem leaves, gathered in the ruins.

Shortly after Julius Caesar established the Roman Empire, Pliny the Elder issued a public complaint: the ever-increasing volume of medicines imported from India was causing a serious drain on the Roman gold treasury.

By that time, medical practitioners on the Indian subcontinent had been studying and documenting the effects of hundreds of botanical compounds for more than 2,500 years. As early explorers traveled to India to trade for gold, silks and spices, carefully compiled Indian medicines were also brought back to Persia, Mesopotamia, Egypt, Greece and Rome.

With the advent of the British, things changed. European colonizer systematically discouraged traditional practices like using neem leaves to protect crops and stored grains and over time, these came to be regarded as "backward". There was a tendency on the part of the colonial rulers to encourage people to abandon their ecologically sound practices in favor of modern chemical products imported from the West. It's only now that efforts are being made to revive the old practices.

To Indians in foreign lands the neem tree brought solace and helped them bridge the gap with their homeland. It symbolized a continuity of tradition and fulfilled the need to live in intimate harmony with nature. Thus the neem tree found itself a new home in Mauritius, Fiji, Australia, East and Sub-Saharan Africa, south East Asia, many countries in Central and South America and Caribbean. With this journey across the oceans, the saga of the neem spread to the far corners of the globe. During Gandhi's Freedom movement there was a renewed interest in things swadeshi, which led to a move to encourage 'swadeshi science'. Neem research in India was a part of this movement.

Pioneering work on commercial use of neem oil and cake was done by the Indian Institute of Science in Bangalore during the 1920s. Until 1933, neem cakes were used in sugarcane fields as a fertilizer and to keep termites at bay. Then pesticides made of synthetic chemicals started appearing in the market and they quickly overshadowed traditional products and methods.

Gandhi, however, kept the tradition of neem alive. He was known to be a firm believer in the goodness of neem. One doctor, in reply to some queries about neem leaves by Gandhi, wrote, "We have made experiments upon neem leaves in our laboratory which revealed that its leaves contain more nutritious elements than any other similar vegetation which had been subjected to chemical analysis earlier." Even leading European forestry experts have now conceded that neem is one of the most promising trees of the 21st century, with a great potential in the fields of pest management, environment protection and medicine.

The most ancient surviving documents that have been translated are the Charaka-Samhita (approximately 500 B.C.) and Susruta Samhita (approximately 300 A.D.). These books have been traced to earlier works dating to 2,000 B.C. and 1,500 B.C. respectively, and the foundation of the Indian system of natural healing, Ayurveda. In these ancient texts neem is mentioned in almost 100 entries for treating a wide range of diseases and symptoms, most of which continue to vex humanity. Long revered for its many healing properties, neem came close to providing a cradle-to-grave health care program and was a part of almost every aspect of life in many parts of the Indian subcontinent upto and including the modern era.

The *Sarira Sthanam* recommended that newborn infants should be anointed with herbs and oil, laid on a silken sheet and fanned with a branch of a neem tree with ample leaves. As the child grew it was given small doses of neem oil when ill and bathed with neem tea to treats cuts, rashes and the lesions of Chicken pox. Daily brushing with neem twigs helped kept both child and adult free of cavities and diseases of the gums.

During adulthood neem bark was burned to make the red ash to be used for religious decoration of the body and neem branches were fanned at the front of religious processions. At the wedding ceremony neem leaves were strewn on the floor of the temple and the air fanned with neem branches. Neem oil lit the night in small lamps. The wood was used to cook the daily meals of beans and grains that had been kept free of insects during storage by mixing them with a light coating of neem oil or by mixing them with neem leaves. Ayurvedic preparations with neem were given for illnesses and neem wood used to make the roof of the house. And at the time of death, neem branches cover the body and neem wood was burned in the funeral pyre.

Neem was so much a part of Indian life that most people were not even conscious of how many ways neem impacted their lives. It has really only been since the dramatic interest in neem by the people of Europe and the United States that they have come to realize the value and significance of neem. A movement to protect the relatively few neem trees in India and the many products given by them is growing as the people of India see the possibility that richer Western nations will create a larger demand for and increase the price of neem products.

To address this potential problem, the Indian government is considering legislation that would ban the export of neem seeds – now regarded as a national treasure – and limit foreign sales to neem oil and manufactured products only.

Chapter **4**

Neem : 'The Village Pharmacy' Goes Global

For centuries, the Neem tree has been known in India as 'Heal all' or 'Sarvarogahari' due to its many and varied healing properties. It has been the most celebrated medicinal plant and finds mention in a number of Puranic texts as also in ancient Persian and Urdu pharmacopoeias who called it a 'Blessed Tree' and the 'Wonder Tree'. It is also called 'Holy Tree' or 'Devine Tree'.

In fact, in ancient times neem was the most celebrated medicinal plant of India and found mention in a number of Puranic texts like the *Atharava Veda, Upanishad, Amarkosha* and *Ghrysutra*. They all dealt with the outstanding qualities of the neem tree as a source of medicine and as a natural pesticide. The great Muslim scholar Ali Gilani called it the 'Blessed Tree' and the ancient Indians called Neem- The 'Village Pharmacy'.

There is growing concern around the world about the increasing use of harmful chemicals in food. Such is the awareness that even in India; it is not unusual to see many progressive farmers keeping a part of their farms free of chemicals for their own consumption. Here they employ the ancient means of farming which include the extensive use of neem tree.

A millennium later, today, neem is once again steadily becoming an agro-scientific celebrity. Of late, it has figured as the priority in seminars and serious agricultural workshops all over the world.

Rediscovery of Neem Tree

The neem tree was rediscovered in 1959 when a German scientist witnessed a locust swarm in Sudan. After the swarm had passed the only tree left untouched by the locusts was a neem tree. On closer investigation it was concluded that the locusts did indeed land on neem trees, but they always left without feeding. Since this discovery, there has been worldwide scientific interest in neem and intense research into its many properties. As a result, we now know that the neem tree contains many natural active ingredients which make it resistant not only to locusts but also to more than three hundred different types of insect, as well as fungi, bacteria, and even viruses. These chemical defences are not only useful in protecting neem trees but can also be used as the basis for natural medicines.

Modern western medicine is finally discovering what the ancient Indians have known for thousands of years: that the neem tree has superb pharmaceutical and pesticide controlling qualities. Its effectiveness, availability and safety have made agro-scientists promote cultivation of neem forests. The azadirachtin compound in neem has been recognized as an effective insecticide that is biologically selective, not harming the useful pest-predators but keeping almost 250 harmful ones at bay.

Neem part and products	Aza content (%)
Neem oil	0.01-0.1
Az-enriched oil	0.1-1.0
Seed Cake	0.005-1.2
Seed Kernels	0.35-0.89
Aqueous extract	0.001-0.02

Neem cake is traditionally put in rice fields as a fertilizer. Scientists recommend coating urea with neem cake to kill nitrifying bacteria. Even water management with neem to control vectors of Japanese encephalitis has shown the victory of neem over DDT.

Rejuvenating Tree

Besides azadirachtin, neem also contains salanin, a chemical substance that is a potent pest controller and is said to be far more effective than the chemically produced diethyl-toluamide that is a part of most of the lethal synthetically produced pesticides. Margosa, the oil extracted from its seeds contains oelic, palmitic and stearic acids as also nimbosterol and tannin. It is the combination of these complex natural substances which makes neem such a rejuvenating tree.

Active ingredients or compounds in neem

Nimbin: anti-inflammatory, anti-pyretic, anti-histamine, anti-fungal

Nimbidin: anti-bacterial, anti-ulcer, analgesic, anti-arrhythmic, anti-fungal

Ninbidol: anti-tubercular, anti-protozoan, anti-pyretic

Gedunin: vasodilator, anti-malarial, anti-fungal

Sodium nimbinate: diuretic, spermicide, anti-arthritic

Quercetin: anti-protozoal

Salannin: insect repellent

Azadirachtin: insect repellent, anti-feedant, anti-hormonal

Neem is also said to aid longevity, guard against heart disease, high blood pressure and arthritis. Besides, it has ingredients which lower cholesterol and clear arteries of fat.

Margosa oil has amazing antiseptic properties as well. It is now being increasingly used in the manufacture of antideratatic soaps and toothpastes. These soaps have natural anti-dandruff qualities. The other uses of margosa oil, the amazing extract from neem, is that it help diabetic patients.

The ancient *vaids* usually recommended a bitter paste of neem leaves and margosa oil as a cure for obesity. Its cosmetic value too is an established Indian tradition as in the old times women applied an application of neem leaves and turmeric paste for a glowing skin.

Uses of various parts of the neem trees

Neem oil is extracted from the seeds of the neem tree and has insecticidal and medicinal properties due to which it has been used for thousands of years in pest control, cosmetics, medicines etc.

Neem seed cake (residue of neem seeds after oil extraction) when used for soil amendment or added to soil, not only enriches the soil with organic matter but also lowers nitrogen losses by inhibiting nitrification. It also works as a nematicide.

Neem leaves are used to treat chickenpox and warts by directly applying to the skin in a paste form or by bathing in water with neem leaves. In order to increase immunity of the body, neem leaves are also taken internally in the form of neem capsules or made into tea. The tea is traditionally taken internally to reduce fever caused by malaria. This tea is extremely bitter. It is also used to soak feet for treating various foot fungi. It has also been reported to work against termites. In Ayurveda, neem leaves are used in curing neuromuscular pains. Neem leaves are also used in storage of grains.

Twigs of neem are also used in India and Africa as toothbrushes. Nowadays toothpastes with neem extracts are also available commercially.

Neem (leaf and seed) extracts have been found to be spermicidal and thus research is being conducted to use neem extracts for making contraceptives. Neem produces pain relieving, anti-inflammatory and fever reducing compounds that can aid in the healing of cuts, burns, earaches, sprains and headaches, as well as fevers.

Neem bark and roots also have medicinal properties. Bark & roots in powdered form are also used to control fleas & ticks on pets.

One of the best-known traditional uses of neem is as nature's toothbrush. Till today, millions of rural folds prefer breaking off a small twig from the neem tree, chewing it until it becomes a soft brush and then rubbing it around the gums and the teeth.

Then, they would split the twig into two and use the flat hard surface as a tongue cleaner. Some old-timers still chew a few leaves of neem every morning as these are said to contain blood-purifying qualities. In the past people applied neem leaves to wounds and sores to hasten healing. Concoctions of neem leaves blended with honey or other soothing herbs are said to cure dermatitis, eczema and other skin rashes. Dried nimbosterol mixed with honey and pepper powder can cure colds, stop bleeding and help a patient suffering from piles.

Medicinal uses for the neem tree

Author/Source	Use	Parts
Shodini, 1997	body heat	leaves
Shodini, 1997	fever	bark
Shodini, 1997	infections	leaves
Shodini, 1997	painful periods	leaves
Shodini, 1997	vaginal problems	bark/leaves
Shodini, 1997	worms	leaves
Sharma, 1996	fever	leaves
Sharma, 1996	haemorrhage	leaves
Sharma, 1996	piles	seeds
Sharma, 1996	wounds	leaves
Sharma, 1996	eye diseases	fruit juice
Sharma, 1996	jaundice	leaves
Sharma, 1996	poisoning	seeds
Sharma, 1996	fumigation	all parts
Sharma, 1996	teeth diseases	root bark
Sharma, 1996	heart diseases	neem decoction
Sharma, 1996	vaginal problems	neem decoction
Sharma, 1996	gray hairs	neem decoction

The medicinal secrets of the neem tree are now coming under the microscope of western doctors. German and American medical scientists, in particular, are carefully researching neem's healing and revitalising properties and concluding that it contains powerful compounds which can act as a potent weapon against a host of illnesses without the side effects linked to most modern miracle drugs in the chemist shop.

The American National Research Council says that neem is "the most promising of all plants which may usher in a completely new era of pest control, provide millions with inexpensive medicines and even reduce the excessive temperature of an overheated globe."

However, it is neem's pest control qualities that have truly stirred the imagination of the western world that discovered this quite by an accident. In 1959 a German agro-scientist, Dr. Heinrich Schmutterer, working on a research project in Sudan, saw a swarm of locusts descend on a farm. They plundered everything except the neem trees. Dr. Schmutterer embarked on an extensive study and his conclusions startled the western scientific community. He discovered that azadirachtin, the complex compound in the neem tree contained potent anti-feedant properties that were repugnant to over 250 species of crop destroying insects. It also retarded the development of larvae thereby decreasing the population of the pests.

Unique Qualities

One of the biggest advantages of the neem is that it is a hardy tree and can take root rapidly even in hostile soil conditions. More than that it does not need too much nourishment and thus it doesn't impinge on the food supply of the other crops. It also has the unique quality of enriching the surrounding soil and making it more conducive for water retention as it contains compounds which neutralise the acidic content in the soil.

Agro scientists say that neem is the most eco-friendly pesticide which nature has bestowed on man. They recommend that neem and its kernel should be liberally mixed with compost and set to rot. The pesticide is ready in around three to four months depending on the weather conditions.

Organic farming using neem as a pesticide is still done on a very miniscule scale in India. There are hardly any pesticide-free farm products available in the country though there is a growing demand for these. However, some companies are claiming to make organic farming a line of their business.

But scientists suggest that rather than switching completely to neem-based organic farming, it may be more practical to switch to what is termed as Integrated Pest Management. This method advocates the judicious use of less harmful chemical pesticides where a natural predator like neem is not effective. This is so because as of now it is practically impossible to switch completely to organic farming as the neem technique works only on a small scale and certain crops require artificially produced pesticides to come to full bloom.

However, many western agro-scientists say that if neem is effective on a small scale, it can be done on a larger scale as well. There is a certain urgency in advocating the use of neem as a pesticide as there is a growing concern on the lethal pesticides being used in our day-to-day foods.

Take for example a commonly used vegetable like okra or bhindi. It is sometimes immersed in a solution of copper sulphate to give it that extra green shine. In fact, a minimum of six to seven chemical pesticides are sprayed on an apple tree before the fruit is plucked. Just before harvesting the apple trees are sprayed with fungicides and pesticides along with daminozide, a growth regulator. Finally the fruit is sprayed with 'alar' to heighten its redness. Once the apples reach the cold storage they are sprayed with pesticides once again to keep off the rats and insects.

If that list makes you dizzy just imagine what it does to your body every time you eat an apple. Which is exactly the reason why scientists are so bullish about the neem option as a pesticide. But not just as a pesticide, neem has its medicinal values as well.

It was as late as 1971 when an American, Robert Larsen, began importing neem to his country. And America, known for its entrepreneurial skills, was quick to cash on the potential. A number of companies in the US began marketing medicines made from neem extract. The most prominent among these is W.R.Grace, a Fortune-500 company, which came out with two products, Margosan-O and Bioneem. The sales of these have been phenomenal.

Suddenly, the exports of the neem seeds from India have ballooned and it is reported that the W.R.Grace company is setting up a plant in India which will process around 7,500 tonnes of neem seeds annually. The result of all the overseas companies rushing to India has also seen a ten-fold rise in the price of neem seeds from Rs. 300 to Rs. 3,000 a tonne.

Ironically, even as the prices shoot up and exports keep rising, the ubiquitous neem may become out of reach for the ordinary Indian farmer. Thus it is imperative that the government simultaneously thinks in terms of subsidies to the agro sector not just to let the neem proliferate but to also let the rich tradition of the neem tree continue.

Experts at the National Botanical Research Institute (NBRI), Lucknow and the erstwhile King George's Medical College (KGMC) here in a joint research have already obtained a patent for a mixture made of Neem bark and roots of a creeper, Tumba, grown in Punjab. They clinically tested the mixture for mouth-cleansing. Dr. C.S. Saimbi, Professor Periodontics, Faculty of Dental Sciences (KGMC) and a researchers' team led by the then Head of Tree Biology division, Dr. H. M. Behl, are behind the success of this formula underlying the mouth-cleansing product. The product awaits marketing by the pharmaceutical industry. This is the first ever Ayurvedic mouthwash anywhere in the world.

Although neem is one of the most ancient and widely used herbs on earth, in-tense scientific investigations into the properties of neem are being undertaken across the globe. These studies verify the efficacy of its traditional uses and re-veal even more uses the plant can be put to. This illustrates again that traditional wisdom can guide modern science in developing remedies for human ailments.

Modern scientists across the world are trying to find even more uses for this remarkable neem tree.

No wonder, Neem in our culture has been ranked higher than Kalpavriksha, the mythological wish-fulfilling tree!

Chapter 5

If Neem Lives......

If neem lives up to its early promise it will help to control many of the world's pests and diseases, as well as reduce erosion, desertification, deforestation, and perhaps even slow the rate of increase in population. So many details remain to be fleshed out, however that is practical possibilities cannot yet be seen even to a limited extent.

The fact that neem is a tree is in some sense a limitation; to mass-produce products on a vast scale from trees is much harder than from annual plants. However, trees also have several advantages. They are perennials that will provide their products for decades, they pose little risk of becoming weeds, and, once established, they require little care. Moreover, growing tree crops these days is an advantage in itself. Indeed, resources harvested from trees are of vital importance to this seriously threatened planet. Reforestation contributes to a better world, and neem is a good candidate for global tree planting.

Whether neem will thrive in dense plantation blocks is not absolutely certain, but there are many sites where it seems ideal. It can grow in certain marginal lands, for example, and therefore does not have to displace food production because it can be raised where soils are too worn out for crops. It even benefits certain types of soils and, like all trees, helps reduce erosion.

Harvesting neem fruits does not destroy the tree; unlike most reforestation species, neem is more profitable standing than felled. Thus, the use of neem products has the merit of promoting a greening of the earth.

GENERAL ACTIONS

Despite some unresolved questions, enough is already known that exploiting certain neem uses can begin immediately. Indeed, the global problems posed by pests, diseases, erosion, deforestation, and desertification are so vast that boldness is called for and some risk is worth taking. This, therefore, is a time for people to bring the plant and its products into international use. An orderly creation of plantations and markets-with reliable availability of uniform, good quality seeds at stable prices could see neem rise steadily to become one of the most widely grown trees in the world perhaps eventually rivaling the African oil palm in its value.

Governments, agencies, and individuals that assist developing nations should support the development of neem plantings, underwrite projects to harvest and process the seeds for use in pest control and assist countries to develop high-quality ecotypes in terms of azadirachtin content and other desirable traits.

In developing neem, there is potential for much innovation. One example is the concept of centering rural industries around neem-extraction facilities. In this system, industrial development would be integrated with neem-tree growing. It might incorporate crops and livestock, but growing neem trees and processing their products would form the core. This integrated combination has a good chance of providing sustainable, self-reliant, and decentralized rural development— a long-sought goal of many economic development programs. In addition, it could help national interests by reducing pesticide imports and perhaps increasing exports.

PESTICIDE RESEARCH

In the coming years, the struggle to keep food out of the jaws of plant-eating pests will increase in importance as human populations increase, living standards rise, demands for quality food (and the consequent emphasis on blemish-free fruits and vegetables) increase, and the public clamour to eliminate synthetic insecticides becomes more insistent. Neem could be the key to opening this new era of safer pest control products and, if so, is likely to be in huge demand.

Although research on neem-based pesticides is under way, it is only a fraction of what it might be. Currently, there are projects in Australia, Bangladesh, Burma, Canada, Dominican Republic, Germany, India, Israel, Kenya, Nigeria, Niger, Mali, Pakistan, and the United States. Nonetheless, most are small, under-supported, and tacked onto other projects. Much greater effort is warranted, and some of the topics for research are discussed below.

Preparation of Extracts

There is now enough information to encourage use of the current formulations. However, "low-tech" methods should be devised to extract and formulate neem materials in ways that can easily be undertaken by farmers who grow their own neem trees for their own use.

At present, the quality of neem extracts varies. The differences seem to depend on the way the seed was handled, stored, or extracted, and perhaps other factors yet to be recognized. Thus, research on the optimal handling of neem materials is particularly needed. Topics to be studied include conditions for storing seed before extraction and before use, as well as the effects of storing and handling the extracts after they have been made. Increasing the storage life of neem formulations is vital.

Before mass-producing neem products for international use, standardization is essential. The efficacy of various batches is impossible to compare now because no standard of potency is being used. An international nomenclature for neem ingredients-perhaps defined in ppm of azadirachtin-would help bring some order out of the current chaos.

Studies of Effectiveness

The potential of neem products as a village-level remedy for the agricultural pests of the tropics should be fully explored. Further research on specific crops and sites, pest organisms, formulations, and application methods is needed.

Modes of Action

Neem derivatives are promising pest control materials, but just how they work on various species is a topic deserving much greater research attention. Basic research to study the effects of neem extracts on hormone regulation and hormone receptors is required.

Formulation of Products

Additional research is also needed to extend the period in which neem products remain active. When sprayed on plants, the extracts are degraded by sunlight within days. As previously noted, one American company has found that retaining a portion of the seed oil and adding an ultraviolet screen extends the activity to several weeks. This, however, relies on industrial ingredients and is covered by a patent. Ways to achieve similar effects in Third World settings are now necessary.

Neem's Predecessor

The public's increasing concern for the environment seems likely to result in a rising demand for pesticides from plants rather than from petroleum. Such "soft" pesticides represent the hope that agricultural pests can be controlled while maintaining environmental stability.

Neem may become a major part of that growth, but it is not the first botanical pesticide. Pyrethrins, which are naturally derived from daisy-like flowers of certain species of Chrysanthemum, have been used for centuries. Almost 2,000 years ago the Chinese knew that chrysanthemum plants had insecticidal value; some 2,400 years ago the Persians used them. Not until recent centuries, however, were the potentials of the pyrethrins, extracted from the flowers, fully appreciated. Supposedly an Armenian trader, who had learned the secret while traveling in the Caucasus, introduced the insecticide into Europe early in the nineteenth century. Last century, Dalmatia (Yugoslavia) became the center of the world's pyrethrum industry, but after World War I, Japan became the main producer. With supplies cut off during World War II, the Allies began producing the flowers in Kenya. Since the 1960s pyrethrum production has been established in the New Guinea highlands also.

Like neem products, pyrethrins are valued for their low toxicity to mammals and birds. However, the ingredients in these insecticidal chrysanthemums are lethal to insects in a different way from those in neem. They are nerve poisons and contact insecticides. Pyrethrum has quick knockdown properties and is the active ingredient in millions of aerosol spray cans people use against flies and mosquitoes.

Despite the development of many synthetic insecticides, this chemical from chrysanthemums has maintained its position as a major commercial product. World production is more than 10,000 tons. Although powerful synthetic analogues have been developed, demand for the natural material has remained high and in the past several years it has been in short supply.

Now neem, another botanical pesticide, can perhaps step up to take an equally important, but complementary, role in the rising soft pesticide market.

Safety

The product Margosan-0® has been tested and certified safe (when used as directed), but more toxicological research on neem extracts is needed. Chronic-exposure tests, higher-mammal studies, and epidemiological evaluations could help identify any potential short- and long-term hazards before massive international use. All in all, appropriate researchers should undertake studies to assess any remaining possibility of toxicity to higher mammals, birds or fish.

Pest Resistance

Because of the complexity of the mixtures and their modes of action, it seems unlikely that any resistance to mixtures of neem products will develop in the short run. However, insects have disproved similar projections with previous pesticides too often for complacency. Neem materials should therefore be used circumspectly. If applied by judicious spot treatments at appropriate times, they may remain effective for centuries. On the other hand, if used indiscriminately in blanket sprays, they may induce resistance in the pests and be rendered ineffective within a few years.

The buildup of resistance is much more likely with refined neem formulations based on a single active ingredient from neem, such as azadirachtin. Pests can probably develop resistance to a single neem ingredient about as readily as to other insecticidal compounds.

Further research into the issue of resistance is called for.

Human Resistance

Recent surveys reveal that in both India and Pakistan most of the poorer farmers mix a handful of neem leaves in their stored grains to protect them from pests. However, the more affluent farmers, although aware of this practice, do not follow it. Some questioned its efficacy, but most did not want to be stigmatized as "backward" for following an ancient and traditional practice. The key to quickly overcoming this misguided attitude is to show that using neem is actually more modern than the modern techniques for which these farmers are paying big money.

Specialized Uses

Many specialized insecticide uses deserve research, especially in tropical areas. One example is neem-based insect-repelling treatments for common products, such as the bags used for holding and shipping food and other perishables.

STRUCTURAL ANALYSIS

Neem materials are a vast storehouse of possible pest-control agents of the future. Azadirachtin, meliantriol, and salannin, for instance, might serve as models for the synthesis of insect-feeding inhibitors and growth regulators for controlling stored-grain pests, grasshoppers, locusts, nematodes, and other pests. Even if such synthetic analogues prove commercially feasible, it is unlikely they will cut greatly into the markets for the directly extracted neem materials.

NEEM OIL RESEARCH

Despite centuries of use in India, neem oil is still poorly understood as compared to palm oil, soybean, and other vegetable oils. Some basic chemistry, as well as processing and product-development research should be most useful.

Oil Purification

The methods used for processing and refining neem fruits and seeds all need improvement. In particular, simple methods that farmers can employ themselves are comparatively inefficient at present. On the other hand, research on the use of advanced separation technology is also required. Problems of deodorizing, refining, and purifying the oil in industrial production has yet to be made practical and economic on a large scale. Modern separation processes, such as selective absorption or high-tech membranes, might prove extremely valuable here.

Neem and the Superbug

As we go to press in December 1991, news is sweeping the nation that a deadly insect infestation has destroyed America's winter melon crop and damaged its lettuce, cabbage, broccoli, cauliflower, and carrot crops. Millions of voracious insects have spread over California's Imperial Valley, massing on the undersides of leaves and sucking plants dry, weakening or killing them in the process. American consumers have been told to expect serious shortages of some fruits and vegetables, not to mention soaring prices.

The poinsettia whitefly, or "superbug" as farmers are calling it, is a new, more potent strain of the sweet potato whitefly (*Bemisia tabaci*). It appears to be pesticide resistant and eats "just about everything" in its path. According to California agriculture experts, asparagus and onions are the only crops that it does not like.

As a result of the tiny fly's attack, California's governor, Pete Wilson, has declared a state of emergency. And no wonder. California farmers have suffered nearly $90 million in damage, more than 2,500 farm workers are out of work, and hundreds of farm-related businesses have had to take huge losses. California's agriculture experts expect that eventually the blizzard-like swarms of tiny flies will destroy $200 million worth of winter vegetables.

What will happen in future years is anybody's guess. California has no native predators that are effective against the superbug, and all the authorized pesticides are largely useless. However, neem is one of the possible answers to the problem. For several years, this very same insect has been one of the prime targets of neem-seed extracts. This was in other parts of the country and on other crops mainly ornamental plants and mainly in greenhouses. There, neem products have controlled the superbug very effectively, but whether they will be the answer to the problem over the vast areas of vegetables and fruits growing in the Imperial Valley is as yet uncertain.

One major problem is that neem is not registered for use on food crops. Another is the lack of supplies of neem seeds. Nonetheless, even the possibility of a natural pesticide for such a knotty problem is cause for hope that a cure can be found.

Product Development

Neem soaps, lubricants, and many other consumer products offer exciting promise, especially for tropical countries. Here, too, there is much scope for invention and product development. Basic needs include formulations, analyses, and standards for quality.

NONINSECT PESTS

Neem opens up many possibilities of new products that could benefit horticulture, silviculture, and agriculture. There is much scope for research and development in this area. It is perhaps not too far-fetched to speculate that the tree's extracts might be employed in the following ways:

- As systemic fungicides for treating sick trees or crops
- For preventatives that could stop fungal diseases from establishing themselves in plants
- In treatments for trees diseased by viruses

- In treatments for crops threatened by garden snails and slugs

HUMAN HEALTH

Studies of neem's medicinal values are urgently needed and include the following topics:

- Effectiveness in alleviating pain or fever.
- Antibacterial and antiviral qualities.
- Control of dental cavities and pyorrhea.
- Use of neem twigs for teeth cleaning in areas where toothpastes are unavailable or beyond the budgets of poor people.
- Topical treatments for lice.
- Use of neem-leaf juice and neem oil in the treatment of psoriasis.
- Topical treatment for warts.
- Treatment for parasites in the human digestive tract.
- Treatment for parasites in the human blood and lymph systems, including those causing malaria, Chagas' disease, river blindness, elephantiasis, and sleeping sickness.

VETERINARY MEDICINE

Under normal use, neem apparently affects a variety of organisms, including bacteria, fungi, molluscs, and protozoan parasites, which may open many avenues for exploratory research in veterinary medicine. Traditionally, Indians have rubbed neem products onto livestock to treat various complaints. Research should be undertaken to confirm the ability of neem oil or neem-seed extracts or a combination of both to repel insects and ticks, as well as to soothe cuts and bruises and to cure scabies. Neem may also help with several serious tropical skin parasites those that cause mange in camels and donkeys, for example.

Neem products should also be tested as a treatment for intestinal parasites, such as roundworms and tapeworms. The oil's efficacy in the treatment of infections, particularly of the genital tract (postpartum inflammations of the uterus, for instance) in animals also deserves attention.

GENETIC IMPROVEMENT

Individual neem trees vary greatly in their morphology and perhaps in their chemical makeup. It is not yet understood whether these differences are based on genetics or environment or both, although it is believed that environmental factors (such as drought stress) play a dominant role. Basic research is needed in this area and will have to be carried out mainly in Asia, where the greatest range of genotypes is to be found.

So far there has been no selection or breeding for maximum pesticide production. One approach is to seek out the trees whose seeds have the highest proportion of azadirachtin. This would have to be done using standardized methods to ensure that differences in seed handling, deterioration and other features do not interfere. A major breakthrough would arise here if the azadirachtin content can be correlated with a visual or readily identified feature of the trees or seedlings. With millions of neems in the world, a rapid qualitative assessment would be most valuable at this time.

The second approach is to select trees that yield maximum numbers of large fruits. The number and weights of fruits on different trees vary greatly, and obtaining the maximum yield of kernels may be economically more important than the per cent of azadirachtin in each kernel.

BIOTECHNOLOGY

Biotechnology research that might benefit neem includes:

- Magnifying desired traits.
- Examining the enzymology and gene expression of limonoid production.
- Transferring neem's pest-resistance genes into agriculturally significant plants.
- Genetically mapping neem's DNA. (This will speed the development of neem products and benefits.)

REFORESTATION

Much valuable research could be done in the area of neem silviculture. This might include assessments of the following:

- Taproot effects.
- Lateral (feeding) root effects.
- Mycorrhizae.
- Other beneficial soil microbes.
- Seed viability (Research is particularly needed to develop methods to extend the period of the viability of neem seeds for replanting).
- Rapid establishment (at present, the horticultural conditions and practices that lead to optimal growth or productions are unknown. Needed are ways to speed up establishment of the trees).
- Provenance selection (selection of genotypes better suited for select sites-relatively dry areas, for instance).

In addition to such silvicultural studies, neem's apparely remarkable ability to survive in cities and to withstand excessive heat, as well as survive air and water pollution should be evaluated. This could well boost its use in urban forestry throughout the tropics.

Wood Products

The possibility of selecting genotypes for the production of various types of wood products should also be examined.

One need is for types with straight trunks and a maximum length of clean bole. These would be used to produce construction lumber.

Another need is for easy-pollarding types suitable for producing building poles. In several countries neem poles are more valued than any other neem products. Genetic selection for optimum branching from a stump cut close to the ground could be helpful here, as could research to determine the best time of the year and the best height at which to cut the trees. Rural producers in Burkina Faso already manage their neems like hedges (*tenkodogo*) to harvest building poles more easily.

Fruit Orchards

Frequent coppicing or pollarding are not conducive to good flowering because they severely restrict the growth of lateral (flower-bearing) branches. This, in turn, reduces the production of fruit. Therefore, to grow neem for its seed and oil requires a different approach.

A neem-fruit plantation of the future will likely consist of trees specially selected for high yields of high oil-bearing seeds and widely spaced to allow for an optimum spread of the lateral branches and an unrestricted formation of the flowers. Producing and managing these plantations has little in common with conventional forestry. Indeed, it is more in the domain of pomology: the art and science of cultivating fruit trees. Sophisticated modern techniques such as clonal selection, tissue culture, pruning, grafting, mulching, and fertilizing with major, minor and trace elements are all research requirements.

Clarification of such features is important. Neem orchards established in this way could provide a regular supply of quality seed and oil and thereby become the basis for a thriving international industry based on neem ingredients.

Agroforestry

By and large, neem appears to be a poor companion for field crops. However, certain plantings might prove suitable for integrating with local farming and grazing practices. Further investigation should be made. Farming systems combining neem, fast-growing timber trees, and shrubs as a combination fallow would likely turn around declining ecosystems of many humid and semiarid tropics while providing a continuing income. Such systems may help restore and maintain soil fertility.

Plant Viruses

In certain old (1920s) experiments it was reported that neem-leaf extracts seemed to overcome viral diseases in beans, tobacco and some other crops. This could prove to be of outstanding importance. On the other hand, the results were inconsistent and there is likelihood that they will prove unrepeatable.

Nonetheless, if neem shows even limited antiviral activity, that alone would be of interest to world agriculture. The fact that its compounds are systemic and that the tree grows in many countries where viruses devastate crops (streak virus in Africa's corn is an example) are additional benefits of possibly enormous consequence. This is a shot in the dark, but worth exploring.

Plant Bacteria

Asians have long used neem to treat bacterial diseases of the skin (see "Medicinal" section), but, at least for now, its use to combat bacterial diseases of plants is a research area wide open for exploration.

RELATED SPECIES

Neem (*Azadirachta indica*) has at least two close relatives, *A. siamensis* and *A. excelsa*. They, too, are promising resources.

A. *siamensis* is known as "edible neem" because its young leaves and flowers contain lower amounts of bitter principles than A. *indica* and are consumed in considerable quantities as a vegetable by people in Burma and Thailand. No negative consequences have been reported. *A. siamensis* also contains azadirachtin in its seed kernels and might be a useful source of pest-control materials as well as food.

A. excelsa is a little-known tree of Southeast Asia. Recently, German researchers have isolated and characterized a new limonoid from its seed kernels. This compound, marrangin, shows the same mode of action as azadirachtin but is two to three times more active. Leaf extracts of *A. excelsa* also show a better efficacy than those of neem itself.

Chapter 6

Neem and Ayurveda

What is Ayurveda?

There are many ways to describe Ayurveda. One could say that it is the medical system of the Gods handed down to man in ancient India. Or one could say simply that it is an ancient system of medicine developed in ancient India. One could also say it is a modern medical system practiced in modern India and all over the world. One could even say that it is more than a medical system that it is an actual way of life. What is so wonderful about Ayurveda is that whatever your perspective it would be correct. Ayurveda is all of these things and more.

Having said that let me give you the most traditional explanation of Ayurveda according to the word itself in the Sanskrit language. The word Ayus or Ayur means life and the word Veda means knowledge or science. So the word Ayurveda means the knowledge of or the science of how to live life. Not just any life but a long and healthy life. Ayurveda accomplishes this because it educates you to understand how everything in the world affects your health and well being. The food you eat, the exercise you perform, the work you do, your mode of transportation, the geographical location you live in, the people you associate with, everything that touches you in life has an effect on your health. What Ayurveda teaches you are how to make not just choices but wise decisions on how to get the quality of life you so richly deserve.

Ayurveda is a Science of Self Healing, because once you know who you are, what your constitution is, and how you get disease imbalances you will be able to make the life style adjustments you need to create the health and longevity you want. A large part of the road back to health is using 'The Amazing Healing Power of Ayurvedic Herbs'.

A History of Ayurveda

Before the advent of writing, the ancient wisdom of this healing system was a part of the spiritual tradition of the Sanatana Dharma (Universal Religion), or Vedic Religion. VedaVyasa, the famous sage, Shaktavesha avatar of Vishnu, put into writing the complete knowledge of Ayurveda, along with the more directly spiritual insights of self realization into a body of scriptural literature called the Vedas and the Vedic literatures.

There were originally four main books of spirituality, which included among other topics, health, astrology, spiritual business, government, army, poetry and spiritual living and behavior. These books are known as the four Vedas; Rig, Sama, Yajur and Atharva.

The Rig Veda, a compilation of verse on the nature of existence, is the oldest surviving book of any Indo-European language (3000 B.C.). The Rig Veda (also known as Rik Veda) refers to the cosmology known as Sankhya which lies at the base of both Ayurveda and Yoga, contains verses on the nature of health and disease, pathogenesis and principles of treatment. Among the Rig Veda are found discussions of the three dosas, Vayu, Pitta and Kapha, and the use of herbs to heal the diseases of the mind and body and to foster longevity. The Atharva Veda lists the eight divisions of Ayurveda: Internal Medicine, Surgery of Head and Neck, Opthamology and Otorinolaryngology, Surgery, Toxicology, Psychiatry, Pediatrics, Gerontology or Science of Rejuvenation, and the Science of Fertility.

The Vedic Sages took the passages from the Vedic Scriptures relating to Ayurveda and compiled separate books dealing only with Ayurveda. One of these books, called the Atreya Samhita is the oldest medical book in the world! The Vedic Brahmanas were not only priests performing religious rites and ceremonies; they also became Vaidyas (physicians of Ayurveda).

The sage-physician- surgeons of the time were the same sages or seers, deeply devoted holy people, who saw health as an integral part of spiritual life. It is said that they received their training of Ayurveda through direct cognition during meditation. In other words, the knowledge of the use of various methods of healing, prevention, longevity and surgery came through Divine revelation; there was no guessing or testing and harming animal. These revelations were transcribed from the oral tradition into book form, interspersed with the other aspects of life and spirituality.

What is fascinating is Ayurveda's use of herbs, foods, aromas, gems, colors, yoga, mantras, lifestyle and surgery. Consequently Ayurveda grew into a respected and widely used system of healing in India. Around 1500 B.C., Ayurveda was delineated into eight specific branches of medicine. There were two main schools of Ayurveda at that time. Atreya- the school of physicians, and Dhanvantari - the school of surgeons. These two schools made Ayurveda a more scientifically verifiable and classifiable medical system.

People from numerous countries came to Indian Ayurvedic schools to learn about this world medicine and the religious scriptures it sprang from. Learned men from China, Tibet, the Greeks, Romans, Egyptians, Afghanistanis, Persians, and more traveled to learn the complete wisdom and bring it back to their own countries. Ayurvedic texts were translated in Arabic and under physicians such as Avicenna and Razi Sempion, both of whom quoted Indian Ayurvedic texts, established Islamic medicine. This style became popular in Europe, and helped to form the foundation of the European tradition in medicine.

In 16th Century Europe, Paracelsus, who is known as the Father of Modern Western Medicine practiced and propagated a system of medicine which borrowed heavily from Ayurveda.There are two main re-organizers of Ayurveda whose works are still existing intact today - Charak and Sushrut. The third major treatise is called the Ashtanga Hridaya, which is a concise version of the works of Charak and Sushrut.

Thus the three main Ayurvedic texts that are still used today are the Charak Samhita (compilation of the oldest book Atreya Samhita), Sushrut Samhita and the Ashtangha Hridaya Samhita.

These books are believed to be over 1,200 years old. It is because these texts still contain the original and complete knowledge of this Ayurvedic world medicine, that Ayurveda is known today as the only complete medical system still in existence. Other forms of medicine from various cultures, although parallel are missing parts of the original information.

Ayurvedic Reference for Neem Use

To open this testimony I will quote from a book entitled 'The Materia Medica of the Hindus' by Uday Chand Dutt, the late civil medical officer of Searampore. It is stated in this book about neem that "This useful tree is indigenous to India and is cultivated all over the country for the sake of its bark, leaves and fruits. These have been used in Hindu medicine from a very remote period. The bark is regarded as bitter, tonic, astringent and useful in fever, thirst, nausea, vomiting and skin diseases. The bitter leaves are used as a pot-herb being made into soup or curry with other vegetables. The slightly aromatic and bitter taste which they impart to the curries thus prepared, is much relished by some. The leaves are moreover an old and popular remedy for skin diseases. The fruits are described as purgative and emollient and useful in intestinal worms, urinary diseases, and ulcers."

It also states in the book that the bark is used in fever; the fresh juice of the leaves is given with salt in intestinal worms, and with honey in jaundice and skin diseases. Neem also enters into several compound preparations used in skin diseases. As an external application to ulcers and skin diseases, neem leaves are used in a variety of forms such as poultice, wash, ointment and liniment. A poultice made of equal parts of neem leaves and sesame seeds are recommended by Chakradatta for unhealthy ulcerations.

In another text 'The Materia Medica of Ayurveda' based on the 'Ayurveda Saukhyam' of Todarananda, by Dr. Bhagwan Dash, neem is mentioned in several places.

- On page 22 it is written: *NIMBA (AZADIRACHTA INDICA A. JUSS.)* Nimba cures aggravated pitta and kapha, chardi (vomiting), vrana (ulcer), hrllasa (nausea) and Kushta (obstinate skin diseases including leprosy). It is cooling, constipative and a digestive stimulant. It cures kasa (coughing), jvara (fever), trt (morbid thirst), krimi (parasitic infection) and meha (obstinant urinary disorders including diabetes)

- On page 329 it is stated that nimba alleviates the vitiation (impurities or corruption) of the blood, pitta and kapha
- On page 420 it is stated that according to Susruta nimba belongs to a group of drugs that can cure daha (burning syndrome) and aruci (anorexia)
- On page 412 it is stated again according to Susruta that nimba belongs to another group of drugs that can alleviate kapha and poisoning, kandu (itching) and cleansing of ulcers
- On page 430 it is stated that the medicated oil which is prepared of nimba is useful for cleansing ulcers

In another book by Dr. Bhagwan Dash 'The Materia Medica of Ayurveda' based on Madanpalas Nighantu, many of the aforementioned qualities of nimba are repeated. However some new information is expressed which I shall now relate.

On page 46 it is mentioned under the section of specific actions that it is constipative. This indicates that along with its anti-bacterial and anti-viral actions it may be useful in dysentery. In a footnote in the same section it has been stated that it suppresses an unsuppurated boil and helps in the bursting open of a suppurated one. In still another statement on specific actions it is mentioned that it is useful for eyes. It appears that they are talking about the leaf for the above mentioned uses, because following these descriptions it lists the attributes, potency and specific action for the fruit of the nimba tree. The attributes are unctuous and light, the potency is hot and the specific action is purgative. As opposed to the leaf which is light in attribute, cold in potency and constipative in its specific action. No other new information is given about neem in this book.

In still another book by Dr. Bhagwan Dash 'A Hand Book of

Ayurveda' in a section on how to manage diabetes he states that taking neem leaves in the morning is good; they reduce blood sugar.

In the now famous western classic on Ayurvedic herbology, 'The Yoga of Herbs', by Drs. Vasant Lad and David Frawley, they outline the qualities and uses of neem in the following manner. First of all they state that the parts used are the bark and leaves not mentioning the fruit or the oil derived from it until later. The energetic are listed as bitter in taste, cooling in its nature and pungent in its post digestive effect on the tissues. The tissues affected are plasma, blood, and fat. The systems affected are the digestive, circulatory, respiratory, and urinary. Its actions on the systems are that of a bitter tonic, antipyretic, alterative, antithelmintic, antiseptic, and antiemetic.

These are the western naturopathic terms for the actions already explained in the above Materia Medicas in Sanskrit. According to Drs. Lad and Frawley, neem is indicated in the following conditions: skin diseases like (urticaria, ringworm, and eczema), parasites, fever, malaria (for which it is famous), cough, thirst, nausea, vomiting, diabetes, tumors, obesity, arthritis, rheumatism, and jaundice.

Precautions are called for in diseases of cold or tissue deficiency. In discussing the preparation of neem they indicate making infusions, decoctions, using the powdered leaf directly, a paste of the fresh leaves, medicated ghee, and medicated oil. The following two paragraphs are direct quotes from the book giving a general explanation of the healing effects of the neem tree.

Neem is one of the most powerful blood-purifiers and detoxifiers in Ayurvedic usage. It cools the fever and clears the toxins involved in most inflammatory skin diseases or those found in ulcerated mucous membranes. It is a powerful febrifuge, effective in malaria and other intermittent and periodic fevers (in which case it is usually used with black pepper and gentian).

Neem can be taken whenever a purification or reduction program is indicated. It clears away all foreign and excess tissue, and possesses a supplementary astringent action that promotes healing. Yet it should be used with discretion where there is severe fatigue or emaciation. In medicated oil, it is one of the best healing and disinfectant agents for skin diseases, and anti-inflammatory agent for joint and muscle pain.

In another book by Dr. Bhagwan Dash "Ayurvedic Cures for Common Diseases" he states that neem is extremely effective for scabies. "The parts of the body affected by scabies should be washed daily with water boiled with neem leaves. Soap prepared with neem oil is very useful. Neem leaves can be chewed and taken internally also. Tender neem leaves which are not very bitter are made into a pill the size of a pea and given to the patient, twice a day."

In still another book by Dr. Bhagwan Dash 'Fundamentals of Ayurvedic Medicine' he points out that in the excavations at Harappa and Mohenjo-Daro in Northern and Western India which date back to 2500 B.C., several therapeutic substances were found including leaves of the neem tree.

We will now start to extract verses from the Charaka Samhita that shed further light on the value and uses of neem.

Charaka Samhita, Sutrasthana:

- In chapter 2 verse 6 neem is recommended for use in the event of gastro-intestinal diseases caused by vitiated kapha and pitta. The physician should prescribe it for emesis being careful not to cause any harm to the body.
- In chapter 3 verse 2 it is stated that neem mixed with several other Indian herbs as well as ox bile and mustard oil will immediately cure obstinate skin diseases including leprosy, leucoderma of recent origin, alopecia, keloids, ringworm, fistula-in-anopiles, cervical adenitis and popular eruptions of human beings. I have not mentioned the names of the other herbs in the formula because two of the herbs are known by their Sanskrit names only and which herb the name identifies is unknown today.
- In chapter 3 verse 8 it is stated that the powder of neem with many other herbs known and unknown all from India when mixed with buttermilk and applied to the body

with an un-named oil would cure pruritus (A medical term for itching). Types include pruritus ani (itching of the skin around the anus) and pruritus vulvae (itching of the external genital area in women), pimples, urticaria, obstinate skin diseases including leprosy and edema.

- In ch.3 vs.14 it is stated that these ten drugs cure pruritis (explanation of pruritis above), neem is one of those drugs and it appears that it could work either by itself or in conjunction with others. The method for administration is not given here.
- In ch.4 vs.9 it is stated that the fresh juice of the neem leaves or a water decoction of them, along with about 12 other herbs in various forms will help rid the body of all diseases due to excessive weight.
- In ch.27 vs.95 neem is said to be an alleviator of kapha and pitta, bitter in taste, cold in potency and pungent in vipak (post digestive effect on the tissues).

Vimanasthana:

- ch.8 vs.150 it states that the flowers of the neem tree help in the elimination of dosas (vata, pitta, kapha) from the head.

Cikitsasathanam:

- ch.3 vs.201 it is stated that neem along with 7 other herbs can cure all five types of fevers as classified in Ayurveda. Vs.203 of the same chapter says the same thing.
- In vs.224 an elaborate formula includes neem and many other herbs, some made into decoctions and some made into fresh paste. These are taken together and boiled in ghee and milk. The medicated ghee thus prepared is an excellent medicine for the cure of fevers, consumption, bronchitis, headache, pain in the sides of the chest, and burning sensation in the scapular region.
- In verse 258 it is stated that neem leaves should be first prepared as a paste, then add double the quantity of water and again the same amount of oil as water. This mixture should be cooked down on a low flame until the wa-

ter is gone (or half the quantity in the pot remains). It is stated that a massage with this medicated oil instantaneously cures fever.

- In verse 307 it is stated that by performing fumigation with the leaves of the neem tree and ghee it will alleviate fever.
- In ch.4 vs.38 it is stated that rakta pitta (bleeding from various parts of the body) can be alleviated by eating neem leaves as a vegetable.
- In ch.5 vs.115 neem prepared with several other herbs, vegetables, and beans mixed with ghee can when consumed by the appropriate patient cure pitta type tumors, fever, morbid thirst, colic pain, giddiness, fainting, and anorexia.
- In ch.6 vs.30 neem mixed with other herbs in decoction form will give relief to patients suffering from pitta diabetes.
- In vs.38 it is said that if neem mixed with other herbs is prepared in oil then it cures kapha diabetes which is secondarily aggravated by vata. If the same mixture of herbs is prepared with ghee it cures pitta diabetes which is secondarily aggravated by vata. If the diabetes is a derangement of all three dosas vata, pitta, and kapha, then all the herbs should be mixed together with ghee and oil cooked and given to the patient.
- In ch.7 vs.43 it is stated that to perform emetic therapy on a person suffering from kustha (obstinate skin diseases including leprosy) on the upper portions of the body one should mix certain fruits and herbs with honey and the juice of neem and other vegetables and drink.
- In vs.47 it says that neem mixed with other herbs and boiled in oil may be administered as a medicated enema in certain conditions.
- In ch.7 vs 57 neem leaves are employed as a brush on dry scaly patches of skin when the patches are numb and devoid of feeling. This will cause a mild bleeding which will drain the corrupt blood from the area and thus aid in healing the stubborn skin disease which is not responding to

treatment otherwise. This procedure is a mild form of bloodletting which is part of the Pancha Karma System (the five cleansings) in Ayurveda.

- In ch.7 vs.65 it is stated that the bark of the neem tree ground into powder should be mixed in equal quantities with many other tree barks, leaves, herbs, and fruits. Then one should add roasted corn flour in a portion of nine times the total amount of the herbs. The patient should then take a dose of this mixture every day with ghee and honey. This is an infallible remedy for the treatment of kustha (obstinate skin diseases including leprosy). It also cures oedema, anemia, leucoderma, sprue syndrome, enlarged inguinal gland, fistula-in-ano, pimples, scabies, and urticarial rash.
- In ch.7 vs.82 it says that the patient suffering from kustha (obstinate skin diseases including leprosy) should take food preparations and medicated ghee prepared by boiling with neem and other herbs.
- In ch.7 vs.97 it says that a decoction of neem can be used as a bath, drink, or massage in treating kustha (skin diseases).
- In ch.7 vs.100 it says that habitual intake of a decoction of neem with other herbs will cure kustha (skin diseases) caused by kapha and pitta. It also says that the medicated ghee prepared from neem will cure kustha caused by vata.
- In vs.101 it also states that neem mixed with a different group of herbs and used in the same way will produce the same results.
- In vs.103 it says that the medicated oil of neem and other herbs mixed together can cure kustha (skin diseases) by applying it externally.
- In vs.112 it is stated that the mixture of a very large quantity of herbs including the bark of the root of the neem tree and its leaves, with mustard oil and cows urine, when massaged into the body of a patient suffering from boils will burst the boils.

- In vs.129 it says that a decoction of neem along with several other herbs is useful for bathing and drinking by a patient suffering from skin diseases.
- In vs.135 it says that if a patient is suffering from a skin disease whose prominant symptoms are bleeding and high pitta then nimbaghrta (neem leaf tea cooked into ghee), should be used by the patient.
- In vs.136 neem with many other herbs should be made into a tea and then cooked into ghee and taken lukewarm internally by people suffering from kustha (skin diseases) caused by vata and pitta, serious gout, fever, burning sensation, abscess, and pustular eruptions.
- In vs.140 it instructs us to use neem as the chief ingredient in a mixture of herbs to be boiled with ghee, and to be used both internally and externally. One great commentator on Ayurvedic texts Gangadhar Sen states that this is the same formula known as nimbaghrta in vs.135.
- In ch.7 vs.157 it says that if a patient with leprosy is losing his fingers and has serious exudations coming from his sores and if maggots are formed in the ulcers, then the patient should be given cow urine, neem and vidanga (in appropriate form) for bath, internal intake, and external application of thick ointment.
- In the following verse no.158 it says that neem with several other herbs mixed together with cow urine should be used for bath, internal intake, and external application for parasitic infection and leprosy.
- In ch.10 vs.32 a recipe is given for a massage oil to be used on epilepsy patients. It is prepared by cooking together the bark of the neem tree with the barks of several other trees in water and adding to 3 parts of that decoction 1 part sesame oil and 1 part goat's urine.
- In ch.12 vs.62 it is said that neem leaves are a useful vegetable for patients suffering from oedema. In vs.72 it is said that by mixing the powder of neem with many other herbs and then mixing that with cow urine you will have a formula good for all types of oedema.

- In ch.14 vs.56 a recipe is given for an ointment for piles. That recipe is made of a paste from elephant bone (probably ivory), neem, and ballataka.
- In ch.14 vs.186 a decoction of neem with other herbs is called for to alleviate bleeding piles. In vs.215 it says to stop bleeding in piles one should make a decoction of neem bark along with other tree barks and wash the affected area.

This ends the information available on neem from Caraka Samhita.

We will now start gathering information from the Susruta Samhita.

- In the section known as Sutrasthanam chapter 36 verse 14 it is said that a medicated oil prepared with neem and other herbs should be mixed with still a different group of herbs to be used for the purpose of purifying the interior of an ulcer.
- In ch.38 vs.4 & 5 it describes how neem and other herbs mixed together destroy the deranged kapham and the effects of poison, and prove beneficial in cases of morbid discharges from the urethra, kustha (skin diseases), fever, vomiting, itching of the body and as a purifying agent in the case of an external ulcer.
- In ch.38 vs.47 neem is described as being part of a group of drugs known as the guduchyadi group after the herb guduchi.
- It states in verse 48 that this group of herbs is used as an appetizer, a general febrifuge, an antidote for nausea, vomiting, thirst and burning sensation in the body.
- In ch.38 vs.61 it is stated that neem belongs to a group of herbs which act as a good vermifuge, and a purifying agent in cases of bad, malignant, or indolent ulcers.
- In ch.43 vs.2 it says that neem should be mixed with madana seeds, honey, and saindhava salt (rock salt mined from the Sindh province formerly in India and now in Pakistan. The equivalent can be obtained in this country from a salt

bed in Utah, the company's name is Orsa salt and the salt is pinkish white because of its unrefined mineral content) to make an emetic.

- In ch.43 vs.6 neem is part of a decoction that is used for lymphatic congestion through emesis.

Susruta Samhita, Cikitsa Sthanam:

- In chapter 1 verses 63, 64, 65, & 66 neem is mentioned in a formula that includes sesame seeds and honey made into a paste. This formula is to be applied when there is a serious infection which has caused a loss of putrid flesh and an ulcerous cavity has formed. The formula is purification for the sores and with the addition of butter it becomes a medicine to heal up the ulcer.
- In chapter 2 verses 64-68 it is said that neem either by itself or in combination with many other herbs could be used for malignant sores or ulcers.
- In ch.6 vs.7&8 it says that for all types of haemorrhoids, the diet should consist of wheat, barley, and rice mixed with ghee, milk and neem soup.
- In ch.8 vs.14 it says to make a plaster of neem leaves and other herbs for the purpose of curing a sinus condition.
- In ch.9 vs.4 it says that mungdal mixed with neem leaves is a wholesome preparation in case of kustha (stubborn skin diseases).
- In ch.9 vs.7 it says that a patient with kaphaja type kustha in the first stages can treat it with a decoction of neem and other herbs cooked in ghee.
- In ch.9 vs.12 it says that in cases of ringworm of the most virulent type neem can be used for baths, plasters, and rubbing.
- In ch.9 vs.31&32 it says that if the patient exhibits the sloughing of putrid flesh, the physician should take old matured mung dal and boil it in a decoction of neem and adding oil give it to the patient as a drink. Where there are worms present in diseased area (in the sores) then a straight decoction of neem should be given to the patient.

- In ch.10 vs.3 it states that certain formulas for leprosy should be administered with a decoction of neem leaf tea sweetened with honey and sugar and acidified with grapes.
- In ch.10 vs.9 a recipe is given for making an avaleha (medicated jelly) out of neem and several other drugs. It appears that the purpose of this jelly is for patients with leprosy.
- In ch.11 vs.6 it recommends using a decoction of neem for a particular type of diabetes known as sura-meha (this is when ones urine has the smell and appearance of alcohol).
- In ch.17 vs.14 neem with sesame is used as a plaster during a sinus operation. The washing of any incidental ulcer is also done with a decoction of neem tea.
- In ch.18 vs.34-36 it is stated that the internal use of a medicated oil of neem with several other drugs always proves efficacious in a case of goitre.
- In ch.19 vs.20 a decoction of the tender leaves of neem and other herbs and the barks of several trees as well as triphala should be used to constantly wash the ulcer on the genital due to kaphaja upadams'a.
- In ch.20 vs.22-23 it states that neem decoction used as an emetic is very useful in clearing pimpies which disfigure the face in youth.
- In ch.20 vs.27 it says that one should cook various herbs in neem oil and use the oil as an application for incidental ulcers that may develop during surgery.
- In ch.22 vs.17 neem decoction is used as a disinfectant wash with other herbs during surgery of the gums.
- In ch.23 vs.16 it states that in case of oedema one should make a decoction of neem and many other herbs and effuse the affected part.
- In ch.24 vs.3 it is stated that of all bitter trees the twig of neem is best of all for brushing the teeth.
- In ch.25 vs.21 there is a recipe for a cosmetic compound consisting of herbs, tree bark, plant stems, and flowers. Neem leaves are an important ingredient in that formula.

It states that the application of that cosmetic imparts a god like effulgence to the complexion of the person using it.

- In ch.37 vs.10 a recipe is given for the reduction of fat, a feeling of physical languor, itches, as well as diseases due to a derangement of kapha. The means of employment is either by snuffing, gargling, drinking, anointing, or enema. The recipe calls for the use of neem and many other herbs.
- In ch.38 vs.17 a recipe is given which is said to speedily conquer an attack of jaundice, diabetes, obesity, impaired digestion, aversion to food, goitre, slow poisoning, elephantiasis, and other diseases due to deranged kapha. The recipe includes neem with many other herbs, and is taken internally.

Susruta Samhita, Sarira Sthanam:

- In this section in chapter 10 verse 20 it is stated that after a child is just born, and has been properly cleansed and massaged with the appropriate herbs and herbal oils she should be laid on a silken sheet and fanned with the branch of a neem tree with ample leaves on it.

Susruta Samhita, Uttar Tantra:

- In this section in chapter 12 verse 10 a recipe is given for making a medicinal ungent stick for the eye and it is used as a post operative application for speedy recovery. In this recipe the resinous exudations of the neem tree itself are used in the preparation.
- In ch.19 vs.13 a recipe has been given for application to a baby's eyes. The disease manifests in the inner lining of the eye, and the symptoms are constant lachrymation and itching with irritation and rubbing the eyes, which are extremely sensitive to sunlight. It seems from the description they are talking about a kind of conjunctivitis. Neem is part of this formula.
- In ch.34 vs.2b it is said that if a child is bothered by Sita-Putana (a goddess who is from the dark side), the physician should take the dung of an owl and a vulture, the cast

off skin of a snake as well as the herbs Ajagandha and Neem leaves and Yashti Madhu (licorice) and use it for fumigating purposes.

- In ch.39 vs.90-94 a recipe for kaphaja fever (with heavy head and much mucus) of neem mixed with many herbs is given.
- In ch.39 vs.103-106 the commentator points out that most texts do not contain this information but it is available in some remote texts so he gives it here as an additional text to verses 103-106. This addition reads "A portion of the decoction of haridra (tumeric), bhadra-musta, tri-phala, neem, etc.,etc., would cure a case of tri-doshaja fever (all three doshas vata, pitta, and kapha, are disturbed at once) with indigestion, water brash, dropsy, cough, and disrelish of food.
- In ch.39 vs.110-111 a recipe is given for Visama jwara (a fever although spontaneous in origin is almost always involved in and intimately connected with either a passing physic condition such as fear, grief, etc. or the presence of any foreign poisonous matter in the system) with symptoms of coming on every fourth day (Chaturthaka jwara). The recipe contains neem and many other herbs. A note: some commentators believe that the herb mentioned here is not neem but musta.
- In ch.39 vs.116 there is a recipe for chronic fever which includes neem and many other herbs.
- In ch.39 vs.117 there is a recipe for scrofula, kustha, fever, ulcers, and diseases of the eyes, ears, nose, and throat, which include neem and many other herbs cooked in ghee.
- In ch.39 vs.124 a recipe is given for rakta-pitta (bleeding from various parts of the body), diseases due to kapha (mucus), perspiration, muco-purulent discharges, atrophy of the limbs, fever, chlorosis (a severe form of iron-deficiency anemia characterized by a yellow green tinge to the skin), erysipelas (an infection of the face caused by streptococcal bacteria, which are thought to enter the skin through a small wound), and scrofula. Neem and many

other herbs are mixed in this formula.

- In ch.39 vs.a recipe of a decoction of neem and jati flowers is prescribed for a fever which is caused by the smell of any herbs or cereals or in one due to the effect of any sort of poison and the aggravated pitta in the system.
- In ch.39 vs.135 it states that when there is a fever whose symptoms are severe burning sensation all over the body, vomiting should be induced by giving a cold infusion of neem leaves with honey and molasses.
- In ch.43 vs.11 it is stated that in the case of kaphaja type of hridroga (heart disease due to too much kapha (mucus), one should induce vomiting with a decoction of neem leaves before starting therapy.
- In ch.48 vs.19 vomiting induced with the help of a draught of the infusion of tender neem leaves taken lukewarm would prove curative in case of kaphaja trishna (a thirst characterized by the constant drinking of water but a craving for more water should be regarded as afflicted with the disease known as trishna (morbid desire for water) in the kaphaja type of trishna the patient does not have an excessive desire for drinking water, but there is some obstruction in the system hence vomiting is the appropriate therapy.
- In ch.61 vs.12-15 it states that in case of insanity due to epilepsy a massage with an oil composed of a decoction of many different herbs and the expressed juices of neem bark with cows urine is the best medicine.

This concludes the entries from the Susruta Samhita in the matter of the various uses of neem.

Chapter 7

Chemistry of Neem

Background

Chemical investigations of neem were undertaken by Indian pharmaceutical chemists in 1919, whereby they isolated acidic principle in neem oil, which they named as 'margosic acid'. However, real chemical research originated in 1942 with isolation of three active constituents, viz., nimbin, nimbidin and nimbinene. In 1963 an Indian scientist extensively examined the chemistry of the active principles of neem. Following the discovery of neem kernel as a locust feeding deterrent, its chemistry has grown considerably. Several compounds have been isolated and characterized. The main feature is that most of them are chemically similar and biogenetically derivable from a tetracyclicterpenes. These are also called liminoids (azadirachtin, meliantrol, salanin etc.) bitter principles and occur in other botanical species as well (Rutaceae and Simaroubaceae). The unraveling of high complex structural features and biogenetic interrelationship represent classic piece of work on natural product chemistry. From the practical side these compounds also exhibit a wide variety of biological activity, for example, pesticides, antifeedants, and cytotoxic properties.

Leaves

Levaes mainly yield quercetin (flavonoid) and nimbosterol (ß-sitosterol) as well as number of liminoids (nimbin and its derivatives). Quercetin (a polyphenolic flavonoid) is known to have antibacterial and antifungal properties. This may perhaps account for the curative properties of leaves for sores and scabies. Limonoids like nimocinolide and isonimocinolide affect fecundity in house flies (*Musca domestica*) at a dose ranging between 100 and 500 ppm. They also show mutagenic properties in mosquitoes (*Aedes aegypti*) producing intermediates. Fresh matured leaves yield an odorous viscous essential oil, which exhibits antifungal activity against fungi (*Trichophyton mentagrophytes*) in vitro. White crystalline flakes obtained from petroleum ether extract of leaves consisting of a mixture of C 14, C 24, C 31 alkanes were found to exceed or equal the lavicidal activity of pyrethrum extract. The principal constituents of neem leave include protein (7.1%), carbohydrates (22.9%), minerals, calcium, phosphorus, vitamin C, carotene etc. But they also contain glutamic acid, tyrosine, aspartic acid, alanine, praline, glutamine and cystine like amino acids, and several fatty acids (dodecanoic, tetradecanoic, elcosanic, etc.).

Flower

Besides, the essential oil consisting of sesquiterpene derivatives, the flowers contain nimbosterol and flavonoids like kaempferol, melicitrin etc. Flowers also yield a waxy material consisting of several fatty acids, viz., behenic (0.7%), arachidic (0.7%), stearic (8.2%), palmitic (13.6%), oleic (6.5%) and linoleic (8.0%). The pollen of neem contains several amino acids like glumatic acid, tyrosine, arginine, methionion, phenylalanine, histidine, arminocaprylic acid and isoleucine.

Bark

The trunk bark contains nimbn (0.04%), nimbinin (0.001%), nimbidin (0.4%), nimbosterol (0.03%), essential oil (0.02%), tannins (6.0%), a bitter principle margosine and 6-desacetyl nimbinene. The stem bark contains tannins (12-16%) and non-tannin (8-11%). The bark contains anti-inflammatory polysaccharide consisting of glucose, arabinose and fructose at a molar ratio 1:1:1 with molecular weight of 8,400. The bark also yields an antitumor polysaccharide. Besides polysaccharides, several diterpenoids, *viz.*, nimbinone, nimbolicin, margocin, nimbidiol, nimbione, etc. have been isolated from stem bark and root bark.

Besides ß- sitosterol, 24-methylenelophenol and nimatone, the heartwood contains, calcium, potassium and iron salts. The heartwood on destructive distillation gives charcoal (30%) and pyroligeneous acid (38.4%). Neem wood contains cellulose, hemicellulose (14.00%) and lignin (14.63%), while wood oil contains ß-sitosterol, cycloeucalenol and 24-methylenecyceloartenol.

The tree exudes a gum, which on hydrolysis yields, L-arabinose, L-fucose, D-galactose and D-glucoronic acid. The older tree exudes a sap containing free sugars (glucose, fructose, mannose and xylose), amino acids (alanine, aminobutyric acid, arginine, asparagines, aspartic acid, glycine, norvaline, praline, etc) and organic acids (citric, malonic, succinic and fumaric). The sap is reported to be useful in the treatment of general weakness and skin diseases.

Seed

Seed is very important both because of its high lipid content as well as the occurrence of a large number of bitter principles (azadirachtin, azadiradione, fraxinellone, nimbin, salannin, salannol, vepinin, vilasinin, etc.) in considerable quantities. Azadirachtin has proven effectiveness as a pesticide against about 200 insect species and is reported as non-toxic to humans.

Neem kernel lipids are similar to the normal glycerides from other oilseeds and contain oleic acid (50-60%), palmitic acid (13-15%), stearic acid (14-19%), linoleic acid (8-16%) and arachidic acid (1-3%). It is brownish yellow, non-drying oil with an acrid taste and unpleasant odour. The quality of the oil differs with the method of processing.

Cake

The composition of neem cake after the extraction of oil varies widely depending on the raw material used for expelling, for example, whole dried fruits, seeds or kernels. The range of the proximate composition in percentage are: crude protein 13-35, carbohydrates 26-50, crude fibre 8-26, fat 2-13, ash 5-18, acid insoluble ash 1-7. The bitter cake has no value as animal or poultry feed. Extraction of cake with 70% alcohol followed by hexane yields a meal free from bitterness and odour, which will be satisfactory as feed. The neem cake is rich in most of the amino acids. It is a potential source of organic manure and contains many plant nutrients, viz., nitrogen 2-3%, phosphorus 1% and potassium 1.4%. It also contains 1.0-1.5% tannic acid and has the highest sulphur content of 1.07 - 1.36% among the oil cakes. The neem cake contains a large number of triterpenoids, more of which are being discovered.

Chapter 8

Home Uses

No other tree can match neem's usefulness. Neem rightfully belongs to the millions of ordinary Indians who learnt to put it to use, as it is this knowledge, passed down through generations, that has helped scientists discover neem's amazing potential. There is no other tree that touches the life and living of such a majority of the country's population.

TIPS ON USING NEEM

- Mix pure dried neem oil with Vaseline in the ratio of 1:5. This combination can be used for repelling insects including mosquitoes as well as for skin disorders, minor cuts, burns, wounds etc.
- For complete skin protection make a strong tea with neem leaves and add to the bath along with a little rose water.
- Boil 10 freshly cleaned neem leaves along with cotton with a litre of water for approx. 10 mins. Cool. Use as an eye-wash in case of conjunctivitis, itching etc.
- For athletes' foot and other foot problems, make a strong tea and soak feet.
- For dandruff and head lice: Massage neem oil mixed with coconut or olive oil into hair and leave for 1 hour. Shampoo. Repeat once weekly for 3 weeks or as long as problem persists.
- To treat a sore throat without antibiotics, gargle with neem leaf water (add 2 - 3 neem leaves to 300 ml water and cool) to which honey has been added.
- For acne, pimples, skin infections pure neem leaf powder mixed with water to the affected area.

- In case of sinusitis, use pure neem oil as nasal drops. Two drops morning and evening.
- Prevent breeding of mosquitoes by adding crushed neem seeds and neem oil to all breeding areas. Neem products ensure complete inhibition of egg laying for seven days.
- Add 30 ml of neem oil to 1 ltr of water. Mix well. Add 1 ml of teepol (liquid detergent) and spray immediately for plant protection. Do not store the mixture; make fresh formulation for each spray.
- Boil 40 - 50 neem leaves in 250 ml of water 20 mins. Cool, strain and refrigerate to use as an astringent.
- Chewing 2 – 3 neem leaves regularly helps purify the blood and in cases of hyperacidity and diabetes.
- To ward of mosquitoes, add 5 - 10% neem oil to any oil and light as a diya (lamp).
- Add shake dried neem leaves for preservation of food grains like rice, wheat, lentils etc. The leaves should be replaced every 2 - 3 months.

Store neem oil in a cool dark place, away from sunlight. In case neem oil solidifies due to low temperatures, put the bottle in warm water (below 95 degree F) to liquefy. Putting the bottle in very hot water may reduce the effectiveness of oil.

COMPONENTS

Since ancient times, neem has been associated with healing in the sub-continent of India. A large number of medicinals, cosmetics, toiletries and pharmaceuticals are now based on neem derivatives because of its unique properties.

Bark:

Neem bark is cool, bitter, astringent, acrid and refrigerant. It is useful in tiredness, cough, fever, loss of appetite, worm infestation. It heals the wounds and is also used in vomiting, skin diseases and excessive thirst.

Leaves:

According to Ayurveda, Neem leaves help in the treatment of

Vatik Disorders (neuro muscular pains). Neem leaves are also reported to remove toxins, purify blood and prevent damage caused by free radical in the body by neutralising them. Neem leaves are reported to be beneficial in eye disorders and insect bite poisons.

Fruits:

Neem fruits are bitter, purgative, antihemorrhodial and anthelmintic in nature.

Flowers:

Neem flowers are used in vitiated conditions of pitta (balancing of the body heat) and kapha (cough formation). They are astringent, anthelmintic and non-toxic.

Seeds:

Neem seeds are also described as anthelminitic, antileprotic, antipoisonous and bitter in taste.

Oil:

Neem oil derived from crushing the seeds is antidermatonic, a powerful anthelmintic and is bitter in taste. It has a wide spectrum of action and is highly medicinal in nature.

Mixture:

Five parts of neem tree i.e. Bark, Root, Fruit, Flower and Leaves together are used in diseases of blood. It is also used in vitiated conditions of excess heat, itching, wound, burning sensation in body and skin diseases.

Following is a informal compilation of some of the investigations done in neem in recent past.

THE LEAF

- Neem leaves are now known to contain nimbin, nimbinene desacetylnimbinase, nimbandial, nimbolide and quercentin.
- Neem leaves have shown potential in the following areas:
- Studies indicate that tender leaves are effective in parasitic infections.

- A 10% aqueous extract of tender leaves has been found to posess anti-viral properties.
- Studies on plasma clotting time using Russel's viper venom have proved that the leaf extract contains a clotting inhibitor. This justifies its use in the treatment of poisonous bites.
- A total extract of Neem leaves has shown potential as a potent Hepatoprotective agent.
- Water extract of Neem leaves have shown significant antiulcer activity.
- Essential oil from fresh leaves has a mild fungicidal action.
- Neem leaf extract shows significant Anti-inflammatory effect.
- Neem leaf extract have shown reduction in the frequency and severity of stress-induced gastric mucosal lesions.
- Intraperitoneal administration of neem leaf, bark and seed extracts revealed immuno-stimulatory properties of neem, which are responsible for their anti-HIV effect.

THE FRUIT & SEEDS

- Azadirachtins from Neem seed kernel, are among more than a 100 compounds found in Neem. So far twelve azadirachtins have been identified, all the twelve have high level of biological activity.
- It has been reported that a single low dose of azadirachtin immunized the kissing bug a transmitter of Chagas disease.
- Azadirachtins have shown inhibition of larval, pupal and adult moults and of reproduction and fitness of both plant-feeding and aquatic larvae like mosquitoes.
- Gedunin, contained in whole fruit has been shown to possess antimalarial activity.

THE BARK

- Nimibidin found in neem bark is now known to be antipyretic and non-irritant, and it has found to be effective in treatment of skin diseases such as eczema, furunculosis, arsenical dermatitis, burn ulcers, Herpes labialis, scabies and seborrhaeic dermatitis.

- It is also effective in the treatment of skin diseases of unknown origin, such as warts and dandruff.
- Extracts of bark have potent diuretic and anti-inflammatory properties.
- Nimbidin and sodium nimbidinate contained in neem bark are reported to possess spermicidal activity.
- Neem bark has shown anti-bacterial activity against various gram positive organisms.

Chapter 9

Body Care

NEEM'S MEDICINAL USES

Medicinal properties of neem have been known to Indians since time immemorial. The earliest Sanskrit medical writings refer to the benefits of neem's fruits, seeds, oil, leaves, roots and bark. Each of these has been used in the Indian Ayurvedic and Unani systems of medicine.

In Ayurvedic literature neem is described in the following manner: 'Neem bark is cool, bitter, astringent, acrid and refrigerant. It is useful in tiredness, cough, fever, loss of appetite, worm infestation. It heals wounds and vitiated conditions of kapha, vomiting, skin diseases, excessive thirst, and diabetes. Neem leaves are reported to be beneficial for eye disorders and insect poisons. It treats Vatik disorder. It is anti-leprotic. It's fruits are bitter, purgative, anti-haemorrhoids and antihelminthic'.

It is claimed that neem provides an answer to many incurable diseases. Traditionally neem products have been used against a wide variety of diseases which include heat-rash, boils, wounds, jaundice, leprosy, skin disorders, stomach ulcers, chicken pox, etc. Modern research also confirms neem's curative powers in case of many diseases and provides indications that neem might in future be used much more widely.

NEEM AND HEALTH

Neem has rightly been called *sarvaroghari*. Since time immemorial, Indians have learnt and made use of neem in a variety of ways both for personal and community health by way of environmental amelioration. Despite all the vicissitudes India has gone through over the centuries, neem has managed to remain a friend, philosopher and guide to an average Indian. It is time this heritage is appreciated and in area of promotional and preventive health care, our indigenous knowledge and resources are made use of on an increasing scale as low-cost, effective ingredient for the realization of the lofty goal of 'Health for all'.

As Naveen Patnaik (1993, p. 40) says, "Possessed of many and great virtues, this native Indian tree has been identified on the five-thousand-year-old seals excavated from the Indus Valley Civilization". How the tradition lives on has also been graphically brought out, "Today the margosa is valued more highly for its capacity to exercise the demon of disease than the spirit of the dead, and an image of the folk goddess Sitala can often be seen suspended from a margosa branch where she guards against small pox, once the great killer of the Indian country side. Renowned for its antiseptic and disinfection properties, the tree is thought to be particularly protective of women and children. Delivery chambers are fumigated with its burning bark (Margosa seed oil has been chemically tested as an external contraceptive, used by women as a spermicide). Dried margosa leaves are burned as mosquito repellent. Fresh leaves, notorious for their bitterness, are cooked and eaten to gain immunity from malaria.

Neem's antiseptic properties are widely recognized now. "Neem preparations are reportedly efficacious against a variety of skin diseases, septic sores, and infected burns. The leaves, applied in the form of poultices or decoctions, are also recommended for boils, ulcers, and eczema. The oil is used for skin diseases such as scrofula, indolent ulcers and ringworm.

Cures for many diseases have been reported but these need to be confirmed independently by trials under controlled conditions. Laboratory tests have shown that neem is effective against certain fungi that infect the human body. Some important fungi against which neem preparations have been found to be effective are: athlete's foot fungus that infects hair, skin and nails; a ringworm that invades both skin and nails of the feet; a fungus of the intestinal tract; a fungus that causes infections of the bronchi, lungs, and mucous membranes and a fungus that is part of the normal mucous flora that can get out of control leading to lesions in mouth (thrush), vagina, skin, hands and lungs.

Neem has been used traditionally in India to treat several viral diseases. Even many medical practitioners believe that smallpox, chicken pox and warts can be treated with a paste of neem leaves - usually rubbed directly on the infected skin. Experiments with smallpox, chicken pox, and fowl pox show that although neem does not cure these diseases, but it is effective for purposes of prevention. 'Crude neem extracts absorb the viruses, effectively preventing them from entering unaffected cells." Recent tests, although unconfirmed, have shown that neem is effective against herpes virus and the viral DNA polymerase of hepatitis B virus. Should these findings be confirmed, neem could be used to cure these dreadful diseases.

Its effectiveness is enhanced on account of its easy and plentiful availability and low cost along with the advantage - a big and critical advantage - of crating income and employment for the poor. Neem is effective against dermatological insects such as maggots and head lice. It is a common practice to apply neem all over the hair to kill head lice.

Rural inhabitants in India and Africa regularly use neem twigs as tooth brushes. Neem twigs contain antiseptic ingredients. That explains how these people are able to maintain healthy teeth and gums. Ayurveda describes neem as herbal drug which is used to clean the teeth and maintain dental hygiene. Neem in the form of powder is also used to brush teeth and massage gums.

Chagas disease is a major health problem in Latin America. It cripples millions of people there. Laboratory tests in Germany and Brazil show that neem may be an answer to this dreadful disease which so far remains largely uncontrollable. The disease is caused by a parasite which is spread by an insect called kissing bug. Extracts of neem have effects on the kissing bugs. Research has shown that 'feeding neem to the bugs not only frees them of parasites, but azadirachtin prevents the young insects from molting and the adults from reproducing'.

In Ayurvedic medicine system neem is used to treat malarial fevers. Recent experiments have shown that one of the neem's components, gedunin (a limonoid), is as effective as quinine against malaria. Malaria affects millions of people and is responsible for about 2 million deaths every year in India and several other countries. China has adopted neem in a big way for its anti-malaria operation. Their formulation "Quinahausa" is going to become available in India as well. Neem oil treated mosquito nets and mosquito-repellent cheap tablets (one paise per tablet) are also becoming popular. Such mosquito nets presently available in the North-East have to be made available in the whole country (Swadeshi Patrika, chaitra-vaishak 2052). Because of growing problems of resistance to conventional treatments, it is becoming more and more difficult to control malaria. Should neem products prove effective cure against malaria, the dream of complete eradication of malaria might become a reality.

Neem is widely used for treating fevers. It has anti-pyretic (fever-reducing) property. In addition, neem products also have analgesic (pain-relieving) and anti-inflammatroy effects, i.e. for most common ailments neem can provide cheap, easily-available and local entrepreneurship medicines.

With revival of interest in Ayurveda as an important, indigenous total health-care system, neem with its therapeutic properties and time-tested usage, more particularly as a household first - aid and safe self-administered medicine as well as a preventative help is bound to stage a big come back.

Dr. Suresh Chaturvedi (1995) has listed the uses of neem in pyrexia, diabetes, urinary problems, filarial, worms, respiratory disorders, dermatological disorders, gynecological disorders and by way of external use for eyes, piles and fistula, wounds, hair, dental hygiene and as fertility regulatory material; in addition to its ophthalmic and toiletries uses. However, there is a need for continued R & D and its transfer to the pharmaceutical industry.

A wide multitude of diseases or conditions can be successfully treated with various elements of neem.

AIDS:

Some of the best news is that neem may help in the search for a prevention or a cure for AIDS. So far, the National Institutes of Health reports encouraging results from in vitro tests for an AIDS prevention and possible cure using extracts from the tree. Professionally administered neem solutions are currently being studied for their effects on cancer, diabetes, heart disease, and AIDS. In 1993, in a preliminary study, the National Institutes of Health reported positive results from in vitro tests where neem bark extracts killed the AIDS virus. Using extracts made by soaking neem bark in water, Dr. Van Der Nat of the Netherlands found that the extract produced a strong immune stimulating reaction. Studies reported in 1992 and 1994 showed neem's ability to enhance the cell-mediated immune response may be used to provide protection from vaginal contraction of the disease if neem is used as a vaginal lubricant preceding intercourse. AIDS may possibly be treated by ingesting neem leaf extracts or the whole leaf or by drinking a neem tea.

Neem contains immune modulating polysaccharide compounds; the polysaccharide may be responsible for increasing antibody production. Other elements of neem may stimulate immune function by enhancing cellular mediated response. This dual action can help the body ward off the frequent infections that generally accompany AIDS.

Arthritis:

Neem has a long history of relieving inflamed joints, supported by recent scientific studies. Most anti-inflammatories, such as aspirin and ibuprofen, irritate the stomach and may be the major cause for upper GI bellding. Ulcers sometimes occur as a result of taking too much of these over-the counter drugs. Neem is comparably effective, anti-inflammatory and does not adversely affect the stomach. The active constituents in its leaves relieve pain by acting on the prostaglandin mechanism and significantly reduce acute derma.

Several studies have shown its usefulness with the disease. Some studies have looked at the ability of neem leaf extracts to reduce inflammation. One suggested that the phenolic compounds containing catechin (which possess anti-inflammatory properties) may produce the anti-inflammatory effects. Another investigation found that quercetin, an antibacterial compound, exists in neem leaves. Other studies have shown that the polysaccharides in neem reduce the inflammation and swelling that occur in arthritis. Not only does neem help reduce inflammation; it also has pain suppressing properties. Neem can also help create a balance in the immune system, directly affecting the progression of arthritis.

Cancer:

Throughout Southeast Asia neem has been used successfully by herbalists for hundreds of years to reduce tumors. Researchers are now supporting these usés. Neem has been tested on many types of cancers, such as skin cancers, using neem-based creams and lymphocytic cancer, using the herb internally. In India, Europe and Japan scientists have found that polysaccharides and liminoids in neem bark, leaves and seed oil reduced tumors and cancers and were effective against lymphocytic leukemia.

In Japan, several issued patents included hot water neem bark extracts; these were effective against several types of cancer. Several extracts were tested at different doses and were compared to standard anticancer agents. Many extracts were equal or better than the standard treatments against solid tumors. Results of tests performed with a more purified extract of the bark produced even better results. Further studies using pure active compounds are hoped to produce even more impressive results.

In another study, one researcher used an extract of neem leaves to prevent the adhesion of cancer cells to other body cells. If cancers can't stick to other cells, the cancer can't spread throughout the body and is more easily destroyed.

Neem's success has been noticeably remarkable with skin cancers. A number of reports have been made by patients that their skin cancers have disappeared after several months of using a neem-based cream on a daily basis. Injections of neem extract around various tumors have shown sizable reduction in a few weeks' time.

Dental Care:

People in both India and Africa have used neem twigs as tooth brushes for centuries. Neem twigs contain antiseptic ingredients necessary for dental hygiene. Neem powder is also used to brush teeth and massage gums.

In Germany many researchers have shown that neem extracts prevent tooth decay and periodontal disease.

Infections, tooth decay, bleeding and sore gums have all been treated successfully with daily use of neem mouth rinse or neem leaf extract added to the water. Some people have reported a total reversal of gum degeneration after using neem for only a few months.

Diabetes:

Because neem is a tonic and a revitalizer, it works effectively in the treatment of diabetes, as well. More than a disease that requires change of diet, diabetes is the leading cause of blindness in people ages twenty-five and seventy-four; it also damages nerves, kidneys, hear and blood vessels; it may even result in the loss of limbs. Incurable, it can be treated in a variety of ways. One recommendation is to take one tablespoon (5ml) of neem leaf juice daily on an empty stomach each morning for three months. An alternative is to chew or take in powder form ten (10) neem leaves daily in the morning. Some studies have shown that oral application of neem leaf extracts reduced a patient's insulin requirements by between 30 and 50 per cent for nonkeytonic, insulin fast and insulin-sensitive diabetes.

Because neem has been found to reduce insulin requirements by upto 50 per cent, without altering blood glucose levels, the Indian Government has approved the sale of neem capsules and tablets through pharmacies and clinics for this purpose. Many of these pills are made of essentially pure, powdered neem leaves.

Karnim, one medication that contains neem and a number of other herbs, available in many countries for treating diabetes, was found to lower blood sugar by more than 50 per cent in twenty weeks and to maintain that level thereafter.

Heart Disease:

Major causes of a heart attack include blood clots, high cholesterol, arrhythmic heart action and high blood pressure. Neem has been helpful in these conditions too. Its leaf extracts have reduced clotting, lowered blood pressure and bad cholesterol, slowed rapid or abnormally high heartbeat and inhibited irregular heart rhythms. Some compounds may produce effects similar to mild sedatives, which reduce anxiety and other emotional or physical states that may prompt a heart attack. The antihistamine effects of the nimbidin in its leaves cause blood vessels to dilate. This may be why the leaves help reduce blood pressure.

A recent study proved that, when a patient took either neem leaf extract or neem capsules for a month, her high cholesterol levels fell subsequently. In another study, alcoholic extract of neem leaves reduced serum cholesterol by approximately 30 per cent two hours after its administration. The cholesterol level stayed low for an additional four hours until testing ceased.

Another study showed that an intravenous alcoholic extract of the leaf produced a large, immediate decrease in blood pressure, lasting for several hours. A neem leaf extract, sodium nimbidinate, given to those with congestive cardiac failure, was successful as a diuretic. Regarding arrthythmic heart action, neem leaf extract exhibited antiarrhythmic activity, which returned to normal within eight minutes of administration.

Malaria:

According to the Neem Association, an international nonprofit organisation, malaria affects hundreds of millions of people worldwide and kills more than two million every year. Malaria is quite common in India and throughout the tropics.

Neem has been shown to be effective in a number of ways against this deadly disease. Both water and alcohol based neem leaf extracts have been confirmed as effective. It has been shown to block the development of the gamete in an infected person.

Neem leaf extract greatly increases the state of oxidationin red blood cells, which prevents normal development of the malaria virus. Irodin A, an active ingredient in the leaves, is toxic to resistant strains of malaris; 100 per cent of the malaria gamete are dead within seventy-two hours with a 1 to 20,000 ratio of active ingredients. Other experiments have used alcoholic extracts of neem leaf, which performed almost as well.

Gedunin and quercetin, compounds found in the leaves, are also effective against malaria. Several studies show that neem extracts are effective even against the more virulent strains of the malaria parasite. Some scientists believe that stimulation of the immune system is a major factor in neem's effectiveness against malaria. The plant also lowers the fever and increases one's appetite, enabling a stronger body to fight the parasite and recover more quickly.

Even though neem may be effective against the parasites that carry malaria, it has not been shown to prevent the malaria infection once it's in the body.

Rheumatism:

Neem leaves have anti-inflammatory activity, similar to that in drugs such as phenyl butazone and cortisone. They can relieve pain and reduce acute pain edema. For rheumatism, tropical applications of a warmed neem cream that contains neem oil and perhaps a mild neem tea will help lessen pain.

Stress:

Relatively new scientific findings indicate that neem may even be useful for reducing anxiety and stress. An experiment was done on test animals to see what, if any effect neem leaf extract had on these conditions. Fresh leaves were crushed and the liquid squeezed out to produce a leaf extract. The extract was given orally to three main sets of animals, in two standard stress tests.

One group received salt water as a base control; another received Valium; another received the neem leaf extract. The third group was subdivided into sets that received ever larger doses. In the elevated plus maze test, doses of neem leaf extract upto 200 mg/kg showed important antianxiety activity equal to or greater than Valium. The test doses of neem leaf extract upto 100 mg/kg were equal to Valium in their antianxiety effect. At 800 mg/kg the effects of the neem totally disappeared. Neem extracts apparently only work in small doses for this application.

The explanation of neem's antianxiety effect may be its ability to increase the amount of serotonin in the brain. Because it works well in small amounts, it could be safer than drugs currently used for stress, which causes many side effects.

Ulcers:

In the Ayurvedic medical tradition, neem is considered a useful therapy for ulcers and gastric discomfort. Compounds in neem have been proven to have antiulcerative effects. Throughout India, people take neem leaves for all sorts of stomach problems. Some scientific evidence exists for its effectiveness for these problems. Peptic ulcers and duodenal ulcers are treated well with neem leaf extracts; nimbidin from seed extracts taken orally prevents duodenal lesions and peptic ulcers, and provides significant reductions in acid output and gastric fluid activity. Low doses of 20 to 40 mg/kg bring the most relief; increased dosages reduce the effectiveness of neem's antiulcerative effects.

Neem is also useful in treating other problems in the stomach and bowels. The herb promotes a healthy digestive system by protecting the stomach, aiding in elimination, and removing toxins and noxious bacteria. Its leaves are often used to treat heartburn and indigestion. Some neem extracts reduce the concentration of hydrochloric acid in the stomach.

Neem extracts are also used to treat gastritis. The extracts reduce the amount of acid in the stomach; their antibacterial and anti-inflammatory properties can relieve the effects of this condition.

Finally, neem has also been shown to be effective for treating digestive disorders such as diarrhoea, dysentery, hyperacidity and constipation. For diarrhoea and dysentery one solution is to take one tablespoon of neem leaf juice with sugar three times a day. For constipation, a neem powder of two or three grams, with three to four black peppers given three times a day is both a laxative and a demulcent.

Vitiligo:

Vitiligo is believed to be an autoimmune disorder that causes patches of skin to lose their color. It occurs in about five per cent of the human population regardless of race, but most commonly in dark-skinned people. The two most common treatments are exposure to sunlight (or PUVA) or corticoster old drugs, but these are not always effective.

Oral doses of neem were tested at least for one year on fifteen patients who had the disease. They also applied a cream made up of several herbs to patched, which were then exposed to the sun. After ninety days, 25 per cent of the patients showed complete relief. No adverse reactions were shown by any participants. Those who stayed on the treatment the longest showed the most improvement. The dosage was four grams of neem leaves three times a day, ideally taken before each meal.

Other studies showed that the internal use of neem leaves and bark were effective even without the cream. It may be possible that neem oil applied to the affected areas could aid in the reversal of discoloration.

Miscellaneous Health Benefits:

Neem truly seems like miraculous natural drug. Neem has been shown to provide an antiviral treatment option for small-pox, chicken-pox, and warts. It is particularly useful for these conditions when applied directly to the skin. This is due in part to its ability to inhibit viruses from multiplying and spreading.

Chronic fatigue is considered to be caused by both viral and fungal infections. Neem, which can attack both, helps the body fight this debilitating syndrome.

Minor cuts, sprains and bruises are treated with neem lotion, cream or leaf extract applied locally. Its anti-inflammatory and antibacterial attributes are soothing to these conditions.

Hepatitis is another disease helped by neem. This often-deadly disease can be transmitted through blood or by ingesting contaminated food or water. Recent studies indicate that neem extracts can block infection by the virus that causes the disease.

Tests in Germany have shown that neem extracts are toxic to the herpes virus and can easily heal cold sores. Both a mild neem leaf tea and a tropical cream application are recommended. Once the eruption has peaked, discontinue the tea (taken after breakfast and after dinner0 and continue to apply cream until the sore has healed.

Chagas disease is a major health problem that infects some sixteen to eighteen million people, with another ninety million at risk in parts of South and Central America. It may be deadly. There is no vaccine and no safe and effective drug for its cure. The disease is caused by a parasite. Trypanosoma cruzi, which is spread by an insect, named the kissing bug.

Lab tests in Germany and Brazil have indicated that neem may be a solution. Neem leaf extracts have negative effects on these pernicious insects. Feeding neem or more specifically a single dose of Azadirachtin to the bugs not only eliminate the parasites, but the Azadirachtin prevents the young from moulting and the adults from reproducing. Neem leaf or seed extracts may also be sprayed throughout the home where the kissing bug lives; this eliminates the parasites and prevents the bugs from laying eggs.

At the moment, scientists are researching the antibacterial and virus-reducing characteristics of the tree. The first studies confirm its effectiveness against selected fungi that occur, for example, on hair (trichophyton), skin and nails (epidermophyton), or in the vagina (candida).

Skin Diseases:

Neem has been highly successfull against harmful fungi, parasites, and viruses. Although it can destroy these, it does not kill off beneficial intestinal flora nor produce adverse side effects. Neem is toxic to several fungi that attack humans, including the causes of athlete's foot and ringworm and candida, which cause yeast infections and thrush. In fact, neem extracts are some of the most powerful Antifungal plant extracts found in the Indian pharmacopia that are used for these conditions. The compounds gedunin and nimbidol, found in the tree's leaves, control the fungi listed above. Basing their studies on the ancient tradition of using neem to purify the air surrounding sick people, two Indian researchers found that neem smoke was successful in suppressing fungal growth and germination.

One of neem's stronger advantages is its effect upon the skin in general. It has been most helpful in treating a variety of skin problems and diseases including psoriasis, eczema and other persistent conditions.

According to a report from the National Research Council's Ad Hoc Panel of the Board on Science and Technology for International Development, neem preparation from the leaves or oils can be used as general antiseptics. Because neem contains antibacterial properties, it is highly effective in treating epidermal conditions such as acne, psoriasis and eczema. It is also used for treating septic sores, infected burns, scrofula, indolent ulcers and ringworm. Stubborn warts can be cleared up when a high-quality neem product is used. Unlike synthetic chemicals that often produce side effects such as rashes, allergic reactions, or redness, neem doesn't seem to create any of these results.

Early Ayurvedic practitioners believed high sugar levels in the body caused skin disease. Neem's bitter quality was considered to counteract the sweetness. Indians historically bathed in neem leaves steeped in hot water. This is still considered a common procedure for curing skin ailments or allergic reactions.

Psoriasis is successfully treated with neem oil. The oil moisturizes and protects the skin while healing the lesions, scaling and irritations. Experiments have shown that patients with psoriasis who have taken neem leaf orally, combined with tropical treatment with neem extracts and neem seed oil, achieve results at least as positive as those who use coal tar and cortisone, the more traditional treatments. Coal tar products are messy and smelly and cortisone can thin the skin when used repeatedly. Neem has neither side effect. It can be used for extended periods of time without any side effects, is easy to apply and is relatively inexpensive.

FUNGICIDES

Neem has proved effective against certain fungi that infect the human body. Such fungi are an increasing problem and have been difficult to control by synthetic fungicides. For example, in one laboratory study, neem preparations showed toxicity to cultures of 14 common fungi, including members of the following genera:

- *Trichophyton*- an "athlete's foot" fungus that infects hair, skin, and nails;
- *Epidermophyton*- a "ringworm" that invades both skin and nails of the feet;
- *Microsporum*- a ringworm that invades hair, skin, and (rarely) nails;
- *Trichosporon*- a fungus of the intestinal tract;
- *Geotrichum*- a yeastlike fungus that causes infections of the bronchi, lungs, and mucous membranes; and
- *Candida*-a yeastlike fungus that is part of the normal mu-

cous flora but can get out of control, leading to lesions in mouth (thrush), vagina, skin, hands, and lungs.

ANTIBACTERIALS

In trials neem oil has suppressed several species of pathogenic bacteria, including:

- *Staphylococcus aureus.* A common source of food poisoning and many pus-forming disorders (for example, boils and abscesses), this bacterium also causes secondary infections in peritonitis, cystitis, and meningitis. Many strains are now resistant to penicillin and other antibiotics, one reason far the widespread occurrence of staphylococcal infections in hospitals.
- *Salmonella typhosa.* This much-feared bacterium, which lives in food and water, causes typhoid, food poisoning, and a variety of infections that include blood poisoning and intestinal inflammation. Current antibiotics are of only uncertain help in treating it.

However, neem has many limitations as an antibiotic. In the latter test, neem showed no antibacterial activity against certain strains of the above bacteria, and none against *Citrobacter, Escherichia coli, Enterobacter, Klebsiella pneumoniae, Proteus mirabilis, Proteus morgasi, Pseudomonas aeruginosa, Pseudomonas EOI, and Streptococcus faecalis.*

ANTIVIRAL AGENTS

In India, there is much interesting, but anecdotal, information attributing antiviral activity to neem. Its efficacy-particularly against pox viruses-is strongly believed, even among those of advanced medical training. Smallpox, chicken pox, and warts have traditionally been treated with a paste of neem leaves-usually rubbed directly onto the infected skin.

Experiments with smallpox, chicken pox, and fowl pox suggest that there may be a true biological basis for this practice. Crude neem extracts absorbed the viruses, effectively preventing them from entering uninfected cells. Unfortunately, no antiviral effects were seen once the infection was established within the cell.

Thus neem was effective prevention, but not cure.

Recent pharmacological studies have supported the belief that neem leaves possess some antiviral activity. So far these are only preliminary and unconfirmed results, but they are intriguing, nonetheless. In the United States, aqueous neem-leaf extracts have shown low to moderate inhibition of the viral DNA polymerase of hepatitis B virus. In Germany, an ethanolic neem-kernel extract has proved effective against herpes virus. And in horticultural studies, crude extracts also seemed to effectively bind certain plant viruses, and so limit infection.

Should these early results prove to be soundly based, an array of extremely virulent and difficult diseases of people-not to mention of wildlife and livestock-might be treated.

LIST OF DISEASES

Medical properties of Neem have been known to Indians since time immemorial. The Neem tree brings joy and freedom from various diseases.

It has proven beneficial or preventative for the following:

Abrasions	Epilepsy	Obesity
Acne	Eczema	Piles
AIDS	Fungal Infections	Peptic Ulcers
Allergies	Fever	Prickly Heat
Arrhythmia	Food Poisoning	Parasites
Arthritis	Genital Warts	Pain
Athletes Foot	Gingivitis	Plague
Amenorrhoea	Gonorrhea	Periodontal Disease
Bed Sores	Gout	Rashes
Birth Control	Gastritis	Rheumatism
Bleeding Gums	Goitre	Sore Throat
Blood Purifier	Gangrene	Sprains
Bronchitis	Heart Disease	Stomach Problems
Bruises	Hemorrhoids	Stress
Burns	Hepatitis	Syphilis
Bad Breath	Herpes	Scabies

Boils & Pimples	High Blood Pressure	Sinusitis
Cavities	Hives	Snake Bite
Chagas Disease	Hypertension	Sores
Chicken Pox	Hair Loss	Smoking
Chlamydia	Heart Burn	Skin Ulcers
Cholesterol	Hangover	Shingles
Chronic Fatigue	Headache	Skin Problems
Circulation (poor)	Influenza	Thrush
Colds	Insomnia	Tuberculosis
Cold Sores	Immune System	Toothache
Cancer	Indigestion	Urinary Tract infection
Conjunctivitis	Intestinal Worms	Urethra Infection
Convulsions	Infected Glands	Ulcers
Cough	Inflammation	Urinary Stones
Cuts	Joint Pains	Viral
Candida	Kidney Problem	Vaginal Disorders
Dental Problems	Lice	Wounds
Diabetes	Leucoderma	Warts
Diaper Rash	Leprosy	Wrinkles
Dry Skin	Measles	Yeast infections
Dandruff	Malaria	Migraines
Earache	Encephalitis	Nausea

Chapter 10

Birth Control

Neem has been shown to be a powerful, relatively inexpensive birth control agent for both men and women. In the first century B.C., Charaka, the Indian physician, gave a detailed method for using neem for contraception. Cotton soaked in neem oil was kept in the vagina for fifteen minutes before intercourse. This killed the sperm.

Research has shown that neem oil acts as a powerful spermicide. This finding is preliminary and may eventually prove of little consequence, but it may also prove of paramount importance. Perhaps 80 per cent of the expected population explosion, which may double the number of people on earth in the next 40 years, will occur in countries where neem can be grown. An inexpensive birth-control method that can be produced in the backyards of ever the remotest and poorest villages could be a vital resource.

Indian scientists have demonstrated that neem oil is a potential new contraceptive for women. Vaginal creams and suppositories made with neem oil are quickly becoming the birth control method of choice in India. When tested against human sperm neem extract (sodium nimbidinate) at 1000 mg was able to kill all sperm in just 5 minutes and required only 30 minutes at a 250 mg level. They are non-irritating and easy to use. It's important to note, however, that even toxic spermicides are not 100 per cent effective. They have the added benefit of preventing vaginal and sexually transmitted diseases. Histopathology failed to reveal any side effects.

Many women in Madagascar chew a handful of neem leaves every day, which according to their statements prevents pregnancies. In the case of unwanted pregnancies, neem is said to be capable of inducing a miscarriage.

Neem has a proven ability to prevent pregnancy. Neem oil has also been shown to work well both before and after sex while some purified extracts only worked before sex as a preventative. Neem oil appears to be the most effective form of neem for birth control, particularly hexane extracted neem oil. After a single injection of a minute amount of neem oil in the uterine horns, a strong cell-mediated immune response reaction produced a long term (up to 12 months) and reversible block in fertility. There were no changes in menstrual cycles or ovarian function.

Neem oil has also been found to prevent implantation and may even have an abortifacient effect similar to pennyroyal, juniper berries, wild ginger, myrrh and angelica. The effects were seen as many as ten days after fertilization in rats though it was most effective at no more than three days. In a study on rats, neem oil was given orally eight to ten days after implantation of the fetus on the uterine wall. In all cases, by day 15, the embryos were all completely resorbed by the body. The animals regained fertility on the next cycle showing no physical problems. Detailed study of the rats revealed increased levels of gamma interferon in the uterus. The neem oil enhanced the local immune response in the uterus. Post coital use of neem oil as birth control does not appear to work by hormonal changes but produces changes in the organs that make pregnancy no longer viable.

Years of study in India by some of the world's leading scientists resulted in the development of a neem-based polyherbal vaginal cream that has both spermicidal and anti-microbial action. The cream combines 25 per cent neem seed extract with extracts from the soap nut and quinine hydrochloride. Based on the success of these experiments, a neem-based contraceptive cream was developed by a pharmaceutical company in India. Tests of its effectiveness showed that it compared favourably with the chemical-based foams and gels. It was safer and easier to use, caused no irritation or discomfort, was nearly 100% effective, and was therefore used more frequently than the foam or gel spermicide. The effect does not appear to be hormonal and is considered a safe and effective alternative to other methods that use hormones.

The studies leading to the development of these products proved that neem oil killed sperm in the vagina within thirty seconds and was effective for up to five hours. Most spermicide creams must be reapplied at least every hour. An important effect of neem oil used in the vagina is that it seems to increase the antigen presenting ability of the uterine tract. This activation of the local immune cell population has a direct spermicidal effect without apparent side effect.

Neem may become the first truly effective birth control "pill" for men. Neem leaf tablets ingested for one month produced reversible male antifertility without affecting sperm production or libido. In India and the United States, exploratory trials show neem extracts reduced fertility in male monkeys without inhibiting libido or sperm production.

In a test of neem's birth control effects with members of the Indian Army, daily oral doses of several drops of neem seed oil in gelatin capsules were given to twenty married soldiers. The effect took six weeks to become 100 percent effective, it remained effective during the entire year of the trial and was reversed six weeks after the subjects stopped taking the capsules. During this time the men experienced no adverse side effects and retained their normal capabilities and desires. There were no pregnancies of any of the wives during the period of the study. This trial was considered so successful that the colonel in charge of the program was honored by the prime minister. A neem-oil formulation called "Sensal" is now sold in India for contraceptive purposes.

For long term birth control for men it appears that a very minute amount of neem oil injected in the vas deferens provides up to eight months of birth control. The tests revealed no obstructions, no change in testosterone production and no anti-sperm antibodies. The local lymph nodes showed increased ability to respond to infections indicating an immune response may be responsible for the birth control effect in men as it is in women.

Neem-leaf extracts have also shown promise as male birth-control products because they reduce fertility in a variety of male mammals. Reportedly, there was no impotence or loss of libido. This shows promise as the first male birth control pill.

Oddly, neem oil has also been taken internally by ascetics who wish to diminish their sexual desire.

Scientists at India's Defence Institute of Physiology and Allied Sciences (DIPAS) have isolated a neem-oil extract (Nim 76) that they believe can be refined into a new birth control method. Their trials have found that neem oil is strongly spermicidal. Rhesus monkey and human spermatozoa, for example, became totally immotile within 30 seconds of contacting the oil.

Studies in 20 rats, 8 rabbits, 14 rhesus monkeys, and 10 human volunteers showed that neem oil applied intravaginally before sexual intercourse prevented pregnancy. Histopathological studies on the rat tissues (vagina, cervix, and uterus) showed no ill effects. By contrast, nonyl-phenoxy polyethoxy ethanol, the spermicide in a popular vaginal contraceptive cream, produced obvious irritation. Radioisotope studies indicated that neem oil was not absorbed from the vagina.

DIPAS scientists maintain that neem oil might be an ideal contraceptive: it is a natural product, readily available, inexpensive, and nontoxic. Moreover, they anticipate that it will be widely accepted. The only disadvantage, they say, is neem oil's unpleasant odor. However, adding a small amount of scent masks most of the smell without reducing the spermicidal property.

All in all, they conclude, neem oil has particular potential for widespread use by the poor. It seems likely to be the cheapest contraceptive available, and villagers in remote areas may well accept it as a regular method of birth control because sophisticated methods are financially beyond their reach and because they are extremely apprehensive about sterilization and other sophisticated methods.

In a scientific article in the Indian Journal of Medical Research, DIPAS researchers report that tests also show that Nim 76 can prevent a fertilized egg from implanting in the wall of the uterus. Nim 76 was effective in rats and rabbits if applied on day 2 to day 7 of the expected pregnancy. The minimum effective dose was very small (only 25 RI for rats). And a month after the applications ceased, the animals were completely fertile again. According to the researchers, there were no deleterious effects on subsequent pregnancies or offspring.

Chapter 11

Economical Potential

INDUSTRIAL USES

Beyond all the possible pesticides and pharmaceuticals, neem provides many useful and valuable common place materials. For instance, oil extracted from the seeds goes into soaps, waxes, and lubricants, as well as into fuels for lighting and heating. The solid residue left after the oil is removed from the kernels is employed as a fertilizer and soil amendment. In addition, wood from the trees is valued for construction, cabinetry, and fuel. The bark is tapped for gum and extracted for tannins and dental-care products. The leaves are sometimes used for emergency livestock feed. And the profuse flowers are a prized source of honey.

Bark:

The bark of the neem tree is considered equal to the leaf in healing properties in the Ayurvedic system. It is used in many preparations to improve general health but is generally known for its marvellous powers of preventing and healing gum diseases and other dental problems. The bark is now known to possess large numbers of catechins and powerful immunemodulatory and immnostimulating compounds.

The bark has been found to contain 3.43% protein, 0.68% alkaloids and 4.16% minerals. The percentage amino acid composition of the total protein generally found by the research was:

- **arginine**-0.125
- **aspargine**-0.375
- **aspartic acid**-0.280

- **cysteine**-0.500
- **glutamic acid**-0.239
- **isonucleicine**-0.057
- **methionine**-0.125
- **norleucine**-0.138
- **phenylalanine**-0.088
- **proline**-0.300
- **tryptophan**-0.456

Some of the other important compounds reported are, nimbin, nimbinin, nimbidin, nimbosterol, and margosine bitter principal.

Polysaccharides in neem bark extracts have been found to possess anti-tumor and interferon enducing as well as anti-inflammatory activities.

Neem bark contains gallic acid, (+)-gallocatechin, (-) epicatechin (as a 2:1 mixture) (+)-catechin and epigallocatechin. These phenolic compounds in the bark are considered to be teh active principals involved in the anti-inflammatory activity. Neem bark increased cellular immunity by the stimulation of the lymphocyte function as shown by an increase in MIF, a lymphokine which, in the body attaches macrophages to monocytes to their sites of action. The immunostimulatory property of neem bark might by the underlying factor in the general stimulating and skin healing properties of neem. Neem bark is also tapped for gum.

Seed:

Neem seed pulp is useful for methane gas production. It is also useful as carbohydrate - rich base for other industrial fermentations.

Neem Oil:

Of all these products, the oil is perhaps the most commercially important. Neem oil contains several compounds which have proven medicinal and agricultural uses of high value. Neem oil is, however, not used generally for these purposes. In composition, it is much like other vegetable oils, composed primarily of triglycerides of oleic, stearic, linoleic, and palmitic acids.

To obtain neem oil, the seeds are first broken open and the kernels separated. The kernels are then pressed in industrial expellers or in hand- or bullock-operated wooden presses (*ghanis*). The oil yield is sometimes as high as 50 per cent of the weight of the kernel. There is vast scope for expanding neem oil production. Collection of neem seeds to be supplied to the crushers can be important means of supplementary employment and income for the poor households, especially the rural women, since the task of seed collection is highly suited to them.

This "cold-pressed oil" is mainly used in lamps, soaps, and other nonedible products. It is generally dark, bitter, and smelly. Unlike most vegetable oils, it contains sulfur compounds, whose pungent odor is reminiscent of garlic.

A large industry in India extracts the oil remaining in the seed cake using hexane. This solvent-extracted oil is not as high quality as the cold-pressed oil, but it also goes into certain soaps and consumer products.

Purifying neem oil is an elaborate and costly process at present. In one method, the smelly sulfur compounds are distilled off, which frees the oil from both odor and susceptibility to rancidity (because it also removes the free fatty acids). This process has long been used industrially.

As an alternative to pressing out the oil, the kernels can be extracted first with alcohol and then with hexane. Alcohol removes the bitter and odoriferous compounds; hexane recovers the oil. This stepwise extraction upgrades both meal and oil. On the other hand, it requires costly solvents and complex facilities. So far, at least, little oil has been produced this way.

Some of the many everyday uses for neem oil in India are discussed below:

Soap

India's supply of neem oil is now used mostly by soap manufacturers. Although much of it goes to small-scale specialty soaps, large-scale producers also use it, mainly because it is cheap. Generally, the crude oil is used to produce coarse laundry soaps. However, more expensive soaps are made by saponifying the crude oil and distilling the resulting fatty acids before adding the lye. The resulting almost colorless and odorless product is suitable for top-quality toilet and laundry soaps.

Cosmetics

Neem is perceived in India as a beauty aid. Powdered leaves, for example, are a major component of at least one widely used facial cream. Purified neem oil is also used in nail polish and other cosmetics.

Lubricants

Neem oil is nondrying, and it resists degradation better than most vegetable oils. In rural India it is commonly used to grease cart wheels. It could find many similar lubrication applications in other locations, especially in village settings in the warmer parts of the world where neem can be grown.

Neem Oil in India

The neem trees occurring throughout India represent a large, although very scattered, resource. Already, neem oil is a common commodity traded freely in the markets, but much more could be produced. It has been estimated that India's neems bear about 3.5 million tons of kernels each year and that, in principle, about 700,000 tons of oil might be recoverable. The annual production in the late 1980s was only around 150,000 tons. (About 34 tons of neem oil were exported in 1990 valued at 300,000 rupees.)

To increase the amount of oil harvested, the Khadi and Village Industries Commission has pioneered various aspects of processing the fruit and seeds over the past two decades. This grass-roots organization located in Pune has been the leading advocate for neem oil as a resource for India's villagers. Already, it has created the makings of a major village industry, developed on a rational and organized basis.

One difficulty, as with most oilseeds of the forest, is that neem must be harvested during the wet season, and without local drying facilities the fruits and seeds rapidly deteriorate and become contaminated with aflatoxin. Ideally, the fruits should be depulped without delay and the seeds thoroughly dried. The Khadi and Village Industries Commission has devised and popularized simple methods for depulping, drying, and decorticating neem products, even in the remotest villages.

FERTILIZERS

Neem has demonstrated considerable potential as a fertilizer. For this purpose, neem cake and neem leaves are especially promising.

Neem Cake

The residue left after the oil has been removed varies widely in composition. However, the broad ranges in composition are:

Crude protein	13-35 per cent
Carbohydrate	26-50 per cent
Crude fibre	8-26 per cent
Fat	2-13 per cent
Ash	5-18 per cent
Acid-insoluble ash	1-17 per cent

This so-called "neem cake" has considerable local potential. Although too bitter for animal feed, it seems to have unique promise as a fertilizer. It contains more nitrogen, phosphorus, potassium, calcium, and magnesium than farmyard manure or sewage sludge. It is widely used in India to fertilize cash crops, particularly sugarcane and vegetables. Ploughed into the soil, it protects plant roots from nematodes and white ants, probably due to its content of the residual limonoids.

Surprisingly, neem cake sometimes seems to make soil more

fertile than calculations predict. This is apparently due to an ingredient that blocks soil bacteria from converting nitrogenous compounds into (useless) nitrogen gas i.e., nitrification. When mixed with urea, before applying in the field, such use of neem coated urea (90:10) can save about 30% of the total chemical nitrogen requirement of crops, which otherwise would go waste and help in reduction the cost of agricultural production.

Neem Leaves:

The cake is not the only source of fertilizer. Neem leaves are not only useful for pest and disease control, they are also fed to livestock mixed with other fodder. In some areas of India's Karnataka State, people grow the tree mainly for its green leaves and twigs, which they "puddle" into flooded rice fields before the rice seedlings are transplanted.

Neem Leaf Ingredients:

- 20 per cent fibre;
- 0 per cent carbohydrates;
- 15 per cent proteins;
- 5 per cent fat;
- 8 per cent ash;
- 2 per cent calcium & contains essential amino acids.

The known amino acid content of the leaf and the percentages are:

- alanine-1.2,
- aspargine-3.4,
- aspartic-2.7,
- cystine-3.3,
- glutamic acid-3.1,
- isoleucine-1.0,
- phenylaline-3.2,
- proline-2.1,
- threonine-2.4,
- tryptophan-1.4,

- taurine-.7,
- valine-2.9.

Neem leaves have been used as mulch in tobacco fields in the Jaffna district of Sri Lanka. In The Gambia, tomato plants matured several weeks earlier and had more numerous and longer branches when mulched with neem leaves. Neem leaves are spread over the plant roots to retain moisture, kill weeds etc. Neem leaves can also be used to protect stored woollen and silk clothes from insects.

TIMBER

As noted previously, neem is a member of the mahogany family, and the properties of its wood resemble mahogany. It is relatively heavy, with a specific gravity varying from 0.56 to 0.85 (average, 0.68). When freshly cut, it has a strong smell. Although easily sawn, worked, polished, and glued, it must be dried carefully because it often splits and warps. It also splits easily when nailed, so that holes must be pre-bored. Nevertheless, it is a good construction timber and is widely used in carts, tool handles, and agricultural implements. In South India it is a common furniture wood.

The heartwood is red when first exposed, but in sunlight it fades to reddish brown. It is aromatic, beautifully mottled, narrowly interlocked, and medium to coarse in texture. It is subject to only slight shrinkage and can be readily worked by hand or machine. Although it lends itself to carving, it does not take a high polish.

The timber is durable even in exposed situations. It is seldom attacked by termites, is resistant to woodworms, and it makes useful fence posts and poles for house construction. Pole wood is especially important in developing countries; the tree's ability to resprout after cutting and to regrow its canopy after pollarding makes neem highly suited to pole production.

FUEL

Neem produces several useful fuels. As mentioned above, its oil is burned in lamps throughout India. In addition, its wood has long been used for firewood. Moreover, the husk from the seeds-containing no oil and representing the bulk of the wastage in pesticide manufacture is mainly employed as fuel.

Because of the tree's good growth and valuable firewood, it has become the most important plantation species in northern Nigeria. It is also grown for fuel around large towns. Charcoal made from this neem wood is of excellent quality, with a calorific value only slightly below that of coal from Nigeria's Enugu mines.

OTHER PRODUCTS

Several products in addition to those previously discussed have been generated from neem. Among them are the following examples.

Resin

An exudate can be "tapped" from the trunk by wounding the bark. This high-protein material is not a substitute for polysaccharide gums, such as "gum arabic". It may, however, have a potential as a food additive, and it is widely used in South Asia as "neem glue."

Bark

Neem bark contains 14 percent tannins, an amount similar to that in conventional tannin-yielding trees (such as *Acacia decurrens*). Moreover, it yields a strong, coarse fibre commonly woven into ropes in the villages of India.

Honey

In parts of Asia neem honey commands premium prices, and people promote apiculture by planting neem trees.

Food

There are odd reports of people eating neem. Leaf teas may be harmful, especially if drunk in quantity over a long period, but it is said that Mahatma Gandhi, who had a hearty respect for the nutritive value of greens, commonly prepared a neem-leaf chutney and ate it with gusto-despite its incredibly bitter taste.

Recently, the discovery of a rare neem tree with "sweet" leaves has been reported.

Fruit pulp

Pericarp represents about half the weight of neem fruits, and when they are processed to obtain the seeds, large quantities of pulp are also produced. This neem-fruit pulp is a promising substrate for generating methane gas, and it may also serve as a carbohydrate-rich base for other industrial fermentations.

ECONOMIC BENEFITS OF NEEM PRODUCTION

- Neem tree has great potential to help small and marginal farmers in rural India, Africa and Latin America. Farmers, who have limited resources, can benefit in many ways from neem. There are easily exploitable, employment and income generation opportunities in the cultivation of neem and processing of neem products, some of which are possible in a decentralized manner on the basis of small investments.
- Most developing countries have vast areas under marginal lands with low productivity. As neem has multiple uses, its crop on marginal lands can make a significant contribution to rural economies.
- There have not been very many studies dealing with economics of neem trees. There are many tangible and intangible costs and returns from the cultivation of neem tree and processing of neem products which need to be estimated through experiments and surveys. One important study in this area is by which tries to estimates costs and benefits.
- In this study, done in the Indian context, the economic felling cycle for Neem is fixed at 23 years. The discount rate used is 12 % per annum. The study takes into account only tangible inputs for and outputs from neem. For inputs, a shadow price factor of 0.80 is used and for outputs a shadows price factor of 1.25 is used. Using data on costs and returns obtained from various published sources, the study provides estimates of benefit-cost (B-C) ration, net

present worth (NPW) and internal rate of return (IRR) from raising one hectare of neem over a felling cycle of 23 years.

- It is hypothetical case of cluster of 5 or 10 neem trees and their economic costs and benefits.
- On the basis of results given in Table III, the authors recommend investment in neem plantation. The net present worth of Rs. 40,838 implies a result in excess of the value of the capital invested plus the specified rate of the return (12%) on that capital invested.

Table No. III

B-C Ratio, NPW and IRR from raising one ha of neem over a felling cycle of 23 years.

I.	B-C Ratio (Rs.)	3.59
II.	NPW (Rs. / ha)	40838
III.	IRR (%)	45.88

Source: Mruthunjaya & Jha, 1993

- It can be seen that the benefit - cost ratio is Rs. 3.59.
- Yet another positive feature of neem plantation is its ability to generate employment. Most of the operations/practices connected with neem plantation and processing are labour intensive. Since NPW is a positive sum (Rs. 40838), B-C ratio is greater than unity (3.59) and IRR is much above the discount rate (48.88 %) investment in neem plantation is recommended as a highly profitable proposition.
- The authors further argue that 'neem plantation can be made much more profitable if efforts are made towards processing of the products from neem. It will only add value to these products but also generate substantial employment in rural sector, e.g..........processing of neem seed through expeller can provide a net income of Rs. 281 per ton'.
- The Arid Forest Research Institute (AFRI), Jodhpur, India are conducting experiments with plantation of neem trees and monitoring its progress in order to work out the timber content and economic viability. They report that very

positive results have been obtained, as per hectare 800 neem trees can be grown and give good timber yield. For the neem age ranging between 15 - 25 years, the timber volume per hectare ranges from over 77 thousands cubic metres to 2.6 lakhs cubic metres. However, since the experimental plantations are still being worked on, more detailed information is awaited.

ECONOMIC POTENTIAL OF NEEM IN THE FUTURE

- According to some estimates, there are about 20 million neem trees in India. This inter-state estimate is slightly less than current estimate of 20 million. A neem tree normally starts fruiting after 3-5 years. In about 10 years it becomes fully productive. Under favourable conditions fresh fruit yield per fully grown tree is about 50 kg per year. If 50% are accessible and tapped, the total neem seed production may well reach the level of 5 million quintals. Present level of collection is far below 50% which shows the potential for additional employment and income generation. If commercial plantation and agro-forestry involving neem in popularized, the potential goes up significantly, with positive and large externalities for pesticides, fertilizers, livestock, dairying and other value-added products.
- Under the optimistic assumption of an azadirachtin content of 5 g per kg of dried kernels there is already in existence reservoir of about 150 tons of azadirachtin per year in India which can be tapped for commercial exploitation. If azadirachtin is to be produced in bulk quantities, 100 kg at least, the fruits must be dried and processed under carefully controlled conditions in order to avoid fungal infection which may cause aflatoxin pollution. With agro-forestry and commercial scale neem plantation, the potential would grow.
- Neem cake seems to be the most economic starting material for production of crude azadirachtin. "One can assume that a standardized crude azadirachtin should be available at around US$ 2 per gram. Only then it can compete with new synthetic insecticides".

- There is a potential of about 5,40,000 tons of seed, which can yield about 1,07,000 tons of oil and 4,25,000 tons of cake. However, in spite of good demand, only about 25 to 30 per cent of the neem seed is collected in India, indicating a large untapped potential. Incentives for neem seed collection-in keeping with the current economic realities-must be strengthened along with organizational improvements for marketing of neem seeds. Organizational, financial inputs and a policy for integrating neem in the framework of agriculture, rural and small industries policies is needed in order to realize this potential.
- Neem production is presently neither attractive nor remunerative. There are several reasons for the lack of interest among farmers. The important reasons are poor yield, deterioration of seeds, lack of information and inadequate marketing facilities which weaken the returns from this activity. Because of poor quality of seeds and their weak bargaining position, the seed collectors get a very low price for their seeds. The price realized by the seed collectors is in the range of Rs. 500 to Rs. 2500 per ton seed, giving total value in the neighbourhood of Rs. 100 crore.
- As a part-time supplementary income, even if a poor villager is able to tap 100 neem trees in a year, an additional income flow of Rs. 10,000 per year can be earned with the modest target of reaching 50% of the tree population. This kind of additional income just by seed collection can be given to one lakh persons. Once can see immense possibilities if neem as a part of agro-forestry is popularized as a part of IRDP and value-added products through village industries.
- Good quality seed would fetch upto Rs. 4000 per ton which doubles our estimated of neem potential.
- The recovery of oil from poor quality seeds is not good. That is why the price paid for such seeds is low. Collection and drying of seeds are the main problems at the village level. The common practice is to broom the ground

under the tree. In the process, dirt gets mixed with the seed. This can be avoided by affecting simple changes in collection process such as spreading gunny mats or those made of local materials or plastic sheets under the tree. These changes cost very little but can help greatly in the collection of clean seeds and improve oil yield.

- The seed needs to be de-pulped immediately after collection, sun dried and stored till crushed for oil extraction. Any delay in de-pulping the seed and drying affects the quality both with respect to oil and azadirachtin content. Properly dried seeds can be stored upto one year, although it has been recommended to store for a minimum of three months after collection for maximum oil recovery.
- Non Government Organizations can play crucial role in formation of seed collector's co-operatives for collection and marketing of neem seeds. This would enable seed collectors to realize better price.
- Adequate supply of good quality neem seeds in a timely fashion is critical for the commercial success of azadirachtin. In India, facilities already exist for extraction of oil from neem seeds. It is possible to use these prexisting facilities for obtaining azadirachtin-rich extracts. However, unlike in the case of oil extraction, to get good quality azadirachtin extracts, the extraction procedures have to be of high standards. Proper care has to be taken in handling seeds at various stages including procurement, drying and storage. If not handled carefully the azadirachtin content in seeds degrades which affects the quality of the azadirachtin formulations.
- One important reason for lack of interest among farmer is that they generally do not consider neem products as a dependable source for plant protection. This is largely due to lack of information. "............. the efforts made so far on the transfer of neem technology are not commensurate with the voluminous data collected on use of neem leaves, seed, kernel, oil, cake, enriched and aqueous formulations of seed kernel and cake, and ready to use neem formula-

tions as insecticides, antifeedants, repellants, growth disruptors, ovipositional repellants and chemosterilants for control of several insect pests on crops and also as nematicides and nitrogen regulators. There is an urgent need to strengthen and gear up to extension wings of State Agriculture Departments and Universities, Krishi Vigyan Kendras, and Research Institutes of ICAR in collaboration with the manufacturers of neem products to disseminate information on neem to farmers.

The best way to popularize the use of neem products is through neem demonstration centres and bridging the gap between labs and farmers. There are many neem products including pesticides which do not require sophisticated technology to produce. This will greatly reduce farmer's dependence on toxic chemical products.

Chapter 12

Veterinary Uses

NEEM IN ANIMAL HEALTH

For centuries neem has been used in India provide health cover to livestock in various forms. It has also very widely been used as animal feed. Ancient Sanskrit literature indicates its applications; as well as afterwards in a large number of indigenous prescriptions and formulations.

Almost every part of the tree is bitter and finds application in indigenous medicine. Records exist that neem has been used in a large number of ailments in animals ranging from systemic disorders to infections and injuries.

In modern veterinary medicine neem extracts are known to possess anti-diabetic, anti-bacterial and anti-viral properties and they have been used successfully in cases of stomach worms and ulcers. The stem and root bark and young fruits are reported to possess astringent, tonic and anti-periodic properties. The root bark is reported to be more active than the stem bark and young fruits. The bark is reported to be beneficial in cutaneous diseases.

SAP:

Some trees, especially near the water courses exude a sap naturally forms the stem-tip. The sap is considered refrigerant, nutrient and tonic, and useful in skin diseases, a tonic in dyspepsia and general debility.

GUM:

The neem bark exudes a clear, bright and amber-coloured gum, known as the East India gum. The gum is stimulant, demulcent and tonic and is useful in catarrhal and other infections.

LEAVES:

The leaves contain nimbin, nimbinene, 6-desacetylnimbiene, nimbandiol, nimbolide and quercetin. The presence of betasitosterol, n-hexacosanol and nonacosane is also reported.

Leaves are carminative and aid digestion. The tender leaves along with *Piper nigrum* Linn., are found to be effective in intestinal helminthiasis. The paste of leaves is useful in ulceration of cow-pox. An aqueous extract (10%) of tender leaves is reported to possess anti-viral properties against vaccinia, variola, foulpox and New Castle disease virus. The extract of leaf yields fractions which marketedly delay the clotting time of blood. The strong decoction of fresh leaves is stated to be an antiseptic. The hot infusion of leaves is used as anodyne for fomenting swollen glands, bruises and sprains.

FRUITS:

The fruit is used as a tonic, antiperiodic, purgative, emollient and as an antithelmintic. The dry fruits are bruised in water and employed to treat cutaneous diseases.

SEED & KERNEL OIL:

The kernels yield a greenish yellow to brown, acrid, bitter fixed oil (40.0-48.9%), known as 'Oil of Margosa.' The oil has many therapeutic uses and is covered in Indian Pharmacopeia. Medicinal properties of the oil are attributed to the presence of bitter principles and odorous compounds. The bitter principles are used in the pharmaceutical industry. Intrauterine medication of oil controls different types of metritis. The oil is reported to have anti-fertility properties. It possesses anti-fungal and antiseptic activity and is found to be active against both Gram negative and Gram positive micro-organisms.

Effect of neem oil has been evaluated in diabetes as antihyperlycaemic agent. The neem oil has shown antihyperglycaemic effect in dogs.

NEEM AS ANIMAL FEED

Leaves:

Neem leaves contain appreciable amount of protein, minerals and carotene and adequate amount of trace minerals except zinc. These may be helpful in alleviating the copper deficiency when feeding straw and dry fodder.

Goat & Camel:

Goat and camel relish lopped neem leaves and quite often these are fed as sole feed to them in winter season when tree is not needed for shed. However, systematic studies are not available on neem feeding by these animals. Keeping in view these animals have the capability to thrive in hot and dry areas, there is considerable scope of rearing them on neem leaves.

Cattle and buffaloes:

The neem leaves have appreciable quantity of digestible crude protein (DCP) and total digestible nutrients (TDN). Cattle can be fed twigs and leaves in small quantities when mixed with other feeds.

Poultry:

Neem oil can be used in poultry rations. The fatty acid composition of oil indicates that it is a rich source of long chain fatty acids. It contains azadirachtin, meliantriol and salannin. Neem oil can be used in poultry rations.

DE-OILED NEEM SEED CAKE IN ANIMAL FEED

This can considerably reduce the shortage of protein supplements in high producing animals. Seeds from neem yield sufficient oil and the residual cake is the major by-product. Neem cake consists of all essential and non-essential amino acids including sulphur containing amino acids but with negligible quantities of valine and tryptophan. The cake contains sulphur 1.07-1.36% which is more than other cakes. The N content varies from 2-3%. The cake has high crude protein, ether extract and fibre contents. Neem seed cake is a very good source of animal protein (up to 40%). The keeping quality is good and it is not easily spoiled on storage nor is it attacked by fungi. The processed cake can be employed as a good poultry feed. Since the cake is bitter, it acts as a good appetizer. It is also a wormicide.

The use of neem in veterinary medicine in India dates back to the times of the epic *Mahabharata* (300 B.C). According to scholars, two of the five Pandava brothers *Nakul* and *Sahadev*, who practiced veterinary medicine, used neem to treat ailing and wounded horses and elephants by applying poultices prepared from neem leaves and neem oil for healing the wounds etc., during the battle of *Mahabharata*. Ancient Sanskrit literature indicates neem applications as feed and in a large number of prescriptions and formulations to provide health cover to livestock in various forms. Various neem preparations were standardized in the form of oils, liniments, powders and liquids. Ayurvedic scholars recommend the use of neem oil as antipyretic, sedative, anti-inflammatory, analgesic, antihistaminic, anthelminthic and as an acaricide.

Neem has been traditionally used against various livestock insects such as maggots, hornflies, blow-flies and biting flies. Neem is also useful for controlling some bacteria of veterinary importance and against intestinal worms in animals. Patnaik, (1993) highlights the livestock friendly medicinal role of neem in the following: "the tree (neem) is revered by Indian herdsmen as a gentle but effective veterinary poultice, a virtue confirmed by the 16th century Portuguese botanist and traveller, Garciada Orta in his "Coloquios".

'Notes on the Bazaar and Indigenous Drugs Useful in the Treatment of Animals' published in 1929, lists the Veterinary applications of Neem in detail. It notes that "leaves, bark and oil expressed from the seeds are generally used. Internally the preparations of the neem tree are a good bitter tonic, antiperiodic and astringent and are used in combination with other drugs having similar properties. They are best administered in the form of a decoction. They are most useful in fever and debility. Externally, the leaves are used in varied forms, such as raw crushed mass, poultice and wash. The bruised leaves, mixed with charcoal or lime, form a good application to wounds, ulcers, pustular eruptions, such as epizootic aphtha, etc. The decoction of the leaves forms a valuable antiseptic and healing lotion to foul sores and ulcers. The leaves boiled with tamarind leaves are applied as a poultice to inflammatory swellings. The oil is applied to wounds as an antiseptic dressing. It is highly efficacious in parasitic diseases, cutaneous affections of all kinds and erysipelas, etc., as it contains sulphur in organic combination. It is also useful in removing maggots from the wounds. The oil is obtained from most of the bazaars". The approx. dosages are also mentioned:

Doses - Bark -		**Doses - Oil**	
Horse	1-2 oz.	Horse	2-4
Cattle	2-3 oz	Cattle	4-6
Sheep	1/4 - 1/2 oz	Sheep	1-2
Dog	1/4 - 1		

Further the Notes contain details on usage, which indicate the widespread acceptance of Neem in Animal Health in India during the early twentieth century.

Neem bark (Margosa), bruised ... 1 oz ... 87 (Drug No.)

Water ... ... 1 pint.

Boil for 20 minutes and strain (DECOCTION). To be given twice daily. A bitter tonic, antiperiodic, and astringent. Doses - Horse and cattle 1/2 - 1 pint; Dog 1-2 oz.

Neem bark (Margosa), bruised ... 1 oz. ... 87 (Drug No.)

Cinnamon (Dalchinni), bruised ... 4 dr. ... 37 (Drug No.)

Cloves (Laung), bruised ... 2 dr. ... 38 (Drug No.)

Water ... ... 1 pint.

Boil for 20 minutes and strain. Given when cold twice daily. A good tonic in debility after an attack of fever. Dose - Horse and Cattle 1/2 - 1 pint; Dog - 1 oz.

Neem or Margosa Oil ... ... 8 oz. ... 87 (Drug No.)

Turpentine (Gandhi-tel) ... ... 4 oz. ... 104 (Drug No.)

Valuable antiseptic application to wounds and ulcers.

Neem or Margosa Oil ... ... 1 pint. ... 87 (Drug No.)

Sulphur (Gundak) ... ... 1 oz. ... 99 (Drug No.)

Mix well. A good liniment for chronic rheumatism. To be well rubbed into the affected part.

In the past few years researchers have been studying ancient prescriptions like Neem with tools of modern bio-chemistry. In a recent trial at an University in Bangalore, it has been observed that alcohol based neem leaf extract showed promising results in vitro trials as compared to other herbs.

Neem leaves and its extracts are being used as immune-stimulants in poultry flocks. In the poultry industry, use of neem leaves is also made to prevent aflatoxicosis caused by *Aspergillus flavus*, which originates from oil cakes or maize, which are not dried properly and used as an ingredient of the feed. Use of neem cake as a protein substitute has an economical advantage in those countries where it is abundant.

Chapter 13

Organic Farming

Organic farming refers to an agricultural production system, wherein plants and crops are grown without the use of any synthetic fertilizers, insecticides, pesticides, fumigants etc. This method of growing crops relies on crop rotation, animal manures and crop residues to ensure high yield and maximum growth of plants and crops. This method also helps to maintain the soil productivity, ensures sufficient supply of nutrients to plant. All organic foods are required to be certified under an organic certification program. Neem has been used for manufacturing many organic products used in agriculture and farming. It is extensively used to grow plants, which lessens the dependence on synthetic products.

The neem tree and its derivatives have great relevance in organic farming practices. This remarkable tree has been identified as a renewable resource for home grown agro-chemicals and nutrients which are bio - degradable, non-toxic and effective.

Long before synthetic chemicals and commercial insecticides and fertilizers were available, neem derivatives were used in Indian villages to protect and nourish crops. Scientific research has shown that neem extracts can influence nearly 400 species of insects.

It is significant that some of these pests are resistant to pesticides, or are inherently difficult to control with conventional pesticides (floral thrips, diamond back moth and several leaf miners). Most neem products belong to the category of medium to broad spectrum pesticides, i.e., they are effective over a wide range of pests.

Using neem derivatives for managing pests is a non-violent approach to controlling pests. Neem products work by intervening at several stages of the insect's life. They may not kill the pest instantaneously but incapacitate it in several ways. Neem very subtly employs effects such as repellence, feeding and ovipositional deterrence, growth inhibition, mating disruption, chemo-sterilization, etc. These are now considered far more desirable than a quick knock-down in integrated pest management programs as they reduce the risk of exposing pests' natural enemies to poisoned food or starvation.

The action of neem products fulfils all priorities among environmental objectives. This unique tree is perhaps the most significant example of how nature can combine diverse functions i.e., the action of de-oiled neem cake as a pesticide cum fertiliser.

Neem Products used in Organic Farming

- Organic pesticides,
- Organic Insecticides,
- Fumigants and sprays,
- Fertilizers,
- Manure,
- Coir,
- Soil Conditioners,
- Repellents,
- Compost,
- Urea coating agent.

Benefits of Using Neem Products in Organic Farming

- Neem products are non toxic,
- Environmental friendly and bio degradable,
- Cheaper than the synthetic products,
- One product can be used for various purposes,
- Increases soil fertility, thus crop yield,
- Can be used for both cash as well as food crops,
- Pests and insects don't develop resistance to neem products.

Chapter **14**

Pest Management

Ecofriendly Natural Pesticide

Pest control, as practiced today in most developing countries relies mainly on the use of imported pesticides. This dependence has to be reduced. Although pesticides are generally profitable on direct crop returns basis, their use often leads to the contamination of terrestrial and aquatic environments, damage to beneficial insects and wild biota, accidental poisoning of humans and livestock, and the twin problems of pest resistance and resurgence.

Scenario of Crop Pest in India

Crop	1920-40		At Present	
	Total Insect Pest	Serious Pest	Total Insect Pest	Serious Pest
Rice	35	10	240	17
Wheat	20	2	100	19
Sugarcane	28	2	240	43
Groundnut	10	4	100	12
Mustard	10	4	38	12
Pulses	35	6	250	34
Cotton	34	9	162	15

More than 500 arthropods pest species have become resistant to one or more insecticides. Resistance of the cotton bollworm, *Helicoverpa armigera*, in India and Pakistan, and of the Colorado potato beetle, *Leptinotarsa decemlineata*, in the USA to all available insecticides, and resistance of the diamondback moth, *Plutella xylostella*, to all classes of insecticides, including *Bacillus thuringiensis*, in Hawaii, Malaysia, the Philippines, Taiwan, and Thailand, illustrates the complexity of the problem. Shifts in pest status-from minor to major, and resurgence of pests, such as white flies, caused by direct or indirect destruction of pest's natural enemies are other unwelcome developments associated with pesticide use.

A World Health Organization and United Nations Environmental Programme report (WHO/UNEP 1989) estimated there are 1 million human pesticide-poisoning cases each year in the world, with about 20,000 deaths, mostly in developing countries. The problem is rendered even more difficult because few, if any, new compounds are coming to replace old insecticides. The cost of developing and registering new pesticides is staggering almost US$ 60 million, and pesticide manufacturers are unwilling to risk investments on products whose market life could be shortened by development of pest resistance.

For ecologically sound, equitable, and ethical pest management, there is a need for control agents that are pest-specific, nontoxic to humans and other biota, biodegradable, less prone to pest resistance and resurgence, and relatively less expensive. Among various options, neem has been identified a source of environmentally "soft" natural pesticides.

Neem has had a long history of use primarily against household and storage pests and to some extent against crop pests in the Indian sub-continent. It was a common practice in rural India to mix dried neem leaves with grains meant for storage. Mixing of neem leave (2-5%) with rice, wheat and other grains is even now practiced in some parts of India and Pakistan. Also, as early as 1930, neem cake was applied to rice and sugarcane fields against stem borers and white ants. Some innovative farmers in Karnataka and Tamil Nadu states in India even today "puddle" green twigs and leaves in rice nursery beds to produce robust seedling and simultaneously ward-off attack by early pests-leafhoppers, plant-hoppers, and whorl maggots.

Controlled experiments confirmed that rice seedlings raised from seed treated with neem kernel extract or cake was vigorous and resistant to rice leafhoppers and plant-hoppers. Early observations that neem leaves were not attacked by swarming locusts were also confirmed in laboratory studies and attributed to neem's antifeedant activity against locusts.

Postharvest losses are notoriously high in developing countries. Worldwide annual losses in store reach up to 10% of all stored grain, i.e. 13 million tons of grain lost due to insects or 100 million tons to failure to store properly. Dr. R.C. Saxena has recently reviewed the potential of neem against pest of stored products grain legumes, maize, sorghum, wheat rice and paddy, potato tubers. At farm level storage and warehouses, the application of neem derivatives to bags and stored grains has provided protection against insect pests. Powdered neem seed kernel mixed with paddy (1 to 2%) significantly reduced infestation and damage to damage to grain during a 3 month storage period; the effectiveness capacity jute bag (100 x 60 cm) controlled 80% of the population of major insects and checked the damage to wheat up to 6 months. The treatment with untreated control. The neem seed extract treatment was as effective as that of 0.0005% primiphos methyl mixed with the grain. Using this technology in Sind, Pakistan, high benefit-cost ratios were obtained by small, medium, and large-scale farmers.

The effectiveness of neem oil alone or in combination with fumigation was evaluated against five major species of stored grain pests infesting rice and paddy grains in a warehouse trials conducted in the Philippines. Rice grain treated with 0.05 to 0.1% neem oil or treated with neem oil after fumigation with 'Phostoxin', and stored for 8 months had significantly less *Tribolium castaneum* adults than in untreated control. Both kinds of neem treatments were as effective as the bag treatment with 'Actellic' at 25ug/cm2 or grain treatment with Actellic at 0.0005%, and suppressed the pest population by 60%. The population build-up also was reduced when either fumigated or non-fumigated rice was stored in bags treated with neem oil at > 1 mg/cm2.

Rhizopertha dominica, Sitophilus oryzae, Oryzaephilus surinmensis, and *Corcyra cephalonica* were similarly affected by neem treatments alone or in combination with prior grain fumigation. Fumigation and Phostoxin were effective only for about 2 months against *R. dominica*, and for up to 6 months against other pest species, while neem oil treatments were effective up to 8 months. Compared with the pest damage to untreated or fumigated rice, neem oil treatment significantly reduced the damage to rice grain. At 8 months after storage, weevil attacked grains in neem treatments were 50% of those in the fumigated rice and 25% of those in the untreated rice. Neem treatments also reduced the pest populations and damage in paddy. In studies conducted in Kenya, the growth and development of 1st instars of the maize weevil, *Sitophilus zeamais*, was completely arrested in maize grain treated with neem oil at 0.02%, while the weight loss of treated cobs was less than 1% as compared with a 50% reduction in weight of untreated cobs stored for 6 months.

While neem treatments cannot replace completely chemical pesticides used in stored products preservation, the amounts of pesticides needed could be reduced, thereby decreasing the pesticide load in food grains. With proper timing and innovative methods of application, their use could be integrated in stored products management.

Ascher and Meisner have reviewed the effects of neem on hematophagous insects affecting humans and livestock. Application of a paste made from neem leaves and turmeric in 4:1 proportion to the skin cured 97% of the patients suffering from scabies caused by the mite *Sarcoptes scabei* in 3-15 d. Monthly sprays of ethanoilic extracts of neem or weekly bathing in azadirachtin-rich aqueous 1:20 'Green Gold' controlled the bush tick, *Ixodes holocylus*, and the cattle tick, *Boophilus microplus* in Australia, but were less effective against the brown dog tick, *Rhipicephalus sanguineus*. In Jamaica, neem kernel extract controlled ticks on cattles and dogs.

Neem products repel and affect the development of mosquitoes. Two percent neem oil mixed in coconut oil, when applied to exposed body parts of human volunteers, provided complete protection for 12 h from bites of all anophelines. Kerosene lamps containing 0.01-1% neem oil, lighted in rooms containing human volunteers, reduced mosquito biting activity as well as catches of mosquitoes resting on walls in the rooms; protection was greater against Anopheles than against Culex.

Effectiveness of mats with neem oil against mosquitoes has also been demonstrated; the vaporizing repelled mosquitoes for 5-7 h at almost negligible cost. The sandfly, *Phleobotumus argentipes*, also was totally repelled by neem oil, mixed with coconut or mustard oil, throughout the night under field conditions in India. Application of neem cake @ 500 kg/ha, either alone or mixed with urea, in paddy fields in southern India reduced the number of pupae of *Culex tritaeniorhynchus*, the vector of Japanese encephalitis, and also resulted in higher grain yield.

What's in a Neem

Neem protects itself from the multitude of pests with a multitude of pesticidal ingredients. Neem seeds and leaves contain many compounds which are useful for pest control. Unlike chemical insecticides, neem compounds work on the insect's hormonal system, not on the digestive or nervous system and therefore doe not lead to development of resistance in future generations. Its main chemical broadside is a mixture of 3 or 4 related compounds, and it backs these up with 20 or so others that are minor but nonetheless active in one way or another. In the main, these compounds belong to a general class of natural products called "triterpenes"; more specifically, "limonoids."

LIMONOIDS

The liminoids present in neem make it a harmless and effective insecticides, pesticide, nematicide, fungicide etc. So far, at least nine neem limonoids have demonstrated an ability to block insect growth, affecting a range of species that includes some of the most deadly pests of agriculture and human health. New limonoids are still being discovered in neem, but azadirachtin, salannin, meliantriol, and nimbin are the best known and, for now at least, seem to be the most significant.

Azadirachtin

One of the first active ingredients isolated from neem, azadirachtin has proved to be the tree's main agent for battling insects. It appears to cause some 90 percent of the effect on most pests. It does not kill insects-at least not immediately. Instead it both repels and disrupts their growth and reproduction. Research over the past 20 years has shown that it is one of the most potent growth regulators and feeding deterrents ever assayed. It will repel or reduce the feeding of many species of pest insects as well as some nematodes. In fact, it is so potent that a mere trace of its presence prevents some insects from even touching plants.

Azadirachtin is structurally similar to insect hormones called "ecdysones," which control the process of metamorphosis as the insects pass from larva to pupa to adult. It affects the corpus cardiacum, an organ similar to the human pituitary, which controls the secretion of hormones. Metamorphosis requires the careful synchrony of many hormones and other physiological changes to be successful, and azadirachtin seems to be an "ecdysone blocker." It blocks the insect's production and release of these vital hormones. Insects then will not molt. This of course breaks their life cycle.

On average, neem kernels contain between 2 and 4 mg of azadirachtin per gram of kernel. The highest figure so far reported- 9 mg per gram measured in samples from Senegal.

Mellantriol

Another feeding inhibitor, meliantriol, is able, in extremely low concentrations, to cause insects to cease eating. The demonstration of its ability to prevent locusts chewing on crops was the first scientific proof for neem's traditional use for insect control on India's crops.

Salannin

Yet a third triterpenoid isolated from neem is salannin. Studies indicate that this compound also powerfully inhibits feeding, but does not influence insect molts. The migratory locust, California red scale, striped cucumber beetle, houseflies, and the Japanese beetle have been strongly deterred in both laboratory and field tests.

Nimbin and Nimbidin

Two more neem components, nimbin and nimbidin, have been found to have antiviral activity. They affect potato virus X, vaccinia virus, and fowl pox virus. They could perhaps open a way to control these and other liral diseases of crops and livestock.

Nimbidin is the primary component of the bitter principles obtained when neem seeds are extracted with alcohol. It occurs in sizable quantities-about 2 percent of the kernel.

Others

Certain minor ingredients also work as antihormones. Research has shown that some of these minor neem chemicals even paralyze the "swallowing mechanism" and so prevent insects from eating. Examples of these newly found limonoids from neem include deacetylazadirachtinol. This ingredient, isolated from fresh fruits, appears to be as effective as azadirachtin in assays against the tobacco budworm, but it has not yet been widely tested in field practice.

Two compounds related to salannin, 3-deacetylsalannin and salannol, recently isolated from neem, also act as antifeedants.

PRODUCTION

Although bioactive compounds are found throughout the tree, those in the seed kernels are the most concentrated and accessible. They are obtained by making various extracts of the kernels and, to a lesser extent, of the press cake. Although the active ingredients are only slightly soluble in water, they are freely soluble in organic solvents such as hydrocarbons, alcohols, ketones or ethers.

No new or unusual technology is required for any of the processing. It can be done using either simple village-scale technology or high technology methods or industrialized facilities. The most common procedures are summarized below.

Water Extraction

The simplest technique (and the most widely employed today) is to crush or grind the kernels and extract them with water. They may, for example, be steeped overnight in a cloth bag suspended in a barrel of water. For reasons not yet understood, this process is less effective than pouring the water into the bag and collecting the extract as it emerges. The resulting crude suspension can be used in the field without further modification. It can also be filtered and employed as a sprayable emulsion.

This is the most promising approach for use in Third World villages. It has been estimated that by using water extraction, 20-30 kg of neem seed can normally treat 1 hectare. At this rate, the annual seed crop from one mature tree could treat up to half a hectare. However, it is necessary to use a lot of water because the active ingredients have very low solubility in water. Normally, the proportions employed are about 500 g of kernel steeped in 10 liters of water.

Water extracts of ground neem leaves are also very useful. Because neem is an evergreen, they are obtainable throughout the year.

Hexane Extraction

If the kernels are grated and steeped in the solvent hexane, only the oil is removed. The oil is not considered an active pesticide. However, new results show that it is an especially interesting material, which in certain cases can be used to kill the eggs of many types of insect, the larvae of mosquitoes, and various stages of certain pests (such as leafhoppers) that are often hard to control by other means.

The residue left after the hexane extraction still contains the main active limonoid ingredients, and subsequent extractions with water or alcohol produce them in large amounts, clean and uncontaminated by oil.

Pentane Extraction

Pentane extracts of seed kernels are effective against spider mites. They reduce the fecundity (number of eggs) of *Tetranychus urticae,* for example. The active principles in the extracts differ from azadirachtin .

Alcohol Extraction

Alcohol extraction is the most direct process for producing neem-based pesticidal materials in concentrated form. Limonoids are highly soluble in alcohol solvents. The grated kernels are usually soaked in ethanol, but sometimes in methanol. The yield of active ingredients varies from 0.2 to 6.2 per cent.

Although water extracts are effective as pesticides, neem compounds are not highly soluble in water; the alcohol extracts are about 50 times more concentrated. They may contain 3.000 parts per million (ppm) or even 100,000 ppm azadirachtin.

FORMULATIONS

As noted, the simplest neem pesticide is a crude extract. However, for more sophisticated use, various modifications can be made. These advanced formulations may convert neem extracts into the form of granules, dust, wettable powders, or emulsifiable concentrates. Aqueous extracts can also be formulated with soap for ease of application against skin diseases.

Other formulations may involve the addition of chemicals or even the chemical modification of the neem ingredients themselves. These changes may be made to increase shelf stability and reproducibility, and for ease of handling or of scaling up the process. They may also reduce phytotoxicity, the damage to sensitive plants.

One particularly valuable class of additives are those that inhibit ultraviolet degradation. These include sesame oil, lecithin, and paraaminobenzoic acid (PABA).

Additives

Mixing neem extracts with other materials can boost their power 10- to 20-fold. Among these so-called "promoters" are sesame oil, pyrethrins (a type of insecticide mostly extracted from chrysanthemum flowers) and piperonyl butoxide. They are used to produce a quicker kill.

Combinations with synthetic pesticides also can work well-they add rapid "knockdown" to neem's ability to suppress the subsequent rebound in the pest population. The effectiveness of neem extracts can even be boosted with the insect-killing Bacillus thuringensis (Bt) to provide a multifaceted pesticide.

METHODS OF APPLICATION

Neem extracts can be applied in many ways, including some of the most sophisticated. For example, they may be employed as sprays, powders, drenches, or diluents in irrigation water-even through trickle- or subsurface-irrigation systems. In addition, they can be applied to plants through injection or topical application, either as dusts or sprays. Moreover, they can be added to baits that attract insects (a process used, for instance, with cockroaches). They are even burned. For example, neem leaves and seeds and dry neem cake are ingredients in some mosquito coils.

SYSTEMIC EFFECT

The fact that the extracts can be taken up by plants (and thereby confer protection from within) is one of neem's most interesting and potentially useful features. As has been noted, however, the level of this systemic activity differs from plant to plant and formulation to formulation. Extracts without oil, with a little oil, and with much oil exhibit different levels of systemic action.

The systemic activity differs with the insect as well. It is not effective on some aphids, for instance. They feed in phloem tissues, where (for reasons yet unknown) the concentration of azadirachtin is very low. Phloem is the plant's outermost layer of conductive tissues and insects such as these, whose mouthparts cannot penetrate past it, are little affected by neem treatments. On the other hand, leafhoppers and planthoppers, that feed at least half the time on the deeper layer of conductive tissues (called the xylem), get knocked down.

Effects on Insects

The growing accumulation of experience demonstrates that neem products work by intervening at several stages of an insect's life. The ingredients from this tree approximate the shape and structure of hormones vital to the lives of insects (not to mention some other invertebrates and even some microbes). The bodies of these insects absorb the neem compounds as if they were the real hormones, but this only blocks their endocrine systems. The resulting deep-seated behavioural and physiological aberrations leave the insects so confused in brain and body that they cannot reproduce and their populations plummet.

Increasingly, approaches of this kind are seen as desirable methods of pest control: pests don't have to be killed instantly if their populations can be incapacitated in ways that are harmless to people and the planet as a whole. In the 1990s this is particularly important: many synthetic pesticides are being withdrawn, few replacements are being registered, and rising numbers of insects are developing resistance to the shrinking number of remaining chemical controls.

The precise effects of the various neem-tree extracts on a given insect species are often difficult to pinpoint. Neem's complexity of ingredients and its mixed modes of action vastly complicate clarification. Moreover, the studies to date are hard to compare because they have used differing test insects, dosages, and formulations. Further, the materials used in various tests have often been handled and stored differently, taken from differing parts of the tree, or produced under different environmental conditions.

But, for all the uncertainty over details, various neem extracts are known to act as various insects in the following ways:

- Disrupting or inhibiting the development of eggs, larvae or pupae.
- Blocking the molting of larvae or nymphs.
- Disrupting mating and sexual communication.

- Repelling larvae and adults.
- Deterring females from laying eggs.
- Sterilizing adults.
- Poisoning larvae and adults.
- Deterring feeding.
- Blocking the ability to "swallow" (that is, reducing the motility of the gut).
- Sending metamorphosis awry at various stages.
- Inhibiting the formation of chitin.

Neem extracts have proved as potent as many commercially available synthetic pesticides. They are effective against dozens of species of insects at concentrations in the parts-per-million range. At present, it can be said that repellency is probably the weakest effect, except in some locust and grasshopper species. Antifeedant activity (although interesting and potentially extremely valuable) is probably of limited significance; its effects are short-lived, and highly variable. Blocking the larvae from molting is likely to be neem's most important quality. Eventually, this larvicidal activity will be used to kill off many pest species.

INSECT AFFECTED

In spite of high selectivity, neem derivatives affect ca. 400 to 500 species of insects belonging to Blattodea, Caelifers, Dermaptera, Diptera, Ensifera, Hetroptera, Hymenoptera, Isoptera, Lepidoptera, Phasmida, Phthiraptera, Siphonoptera and Thysanoptera, one species of ostracad, several species of mites, and nematodes and even noxious snails and fungi, including aflatoxin-producing *Aspergillus flavus*. Results of field trials in some major food crops in tropical countries will illustrate the value of neem based pest management for enhancing agricultural productivity in Asia and Africa.

In general, it can be said that neem products are medium- to broad-spectrum pesticides of plant-eating (phytophagous) insects. They affect members of most, if not all, orders of insects, including those discussed below.

Orthoptera

In Orthoptera (such as grasshoppers, crickets, locusts), the antifeedant effect seems especially important. A number of species refuse to feed on neem-treated plants for several days, sometimes several weeks. Recently, a new effect, which converts the desert locust from the gregarious swarming form into its nonmarauding solitary form, has been discovered.

Homoptera

Aphids, leafhoppers, psyllids, whiteflies, scale insects, and other homopterous pests are sensitive to neem products to varying degrees. For instance, nymphs of leafhoppers and planthoppers show considerable antifeedant and growth-regulating effects. However, scale insects (especially soft scale), are little affected. Phloem feeders, such as aphids, are in general not good candidates for neem used systemically (see earlier). In some cases, the host plant may influence the degree of control; this seems to apply to some whiteflies, which are affected on some crops but not on others.

Neem derivatives may also influence the ability of homopterous insects to carry and transmit certain viruses. It has been shown, for example, that low doses keep the green fice leafhopper from infecting rice fields with tungro virus. The cause is uncertain but seems to be only partly owing to neem killing the insects or modifying their feeding behaviour.

Thysanoptera

Neem is very effective on thrips larvae, which occur in the soil. However, once the adult thrips and related pests have taken up residence on the plants themselves, they are less sensitive to neem extracts. Oily formulations have shown some success in exploratory trials (perhaps because the oil coated and suffocated these minute creatures).

Coleoptera

The larvae of all kinds of beetles—especially those of phytophagous coccinellids (Mexican bean beetle and cucumber beetle, for example) and chrysomelids (Colorado potato beetle and others)-are also sensitive to neem products. They refuse to feed on neem-treated plants, they grow slowly, and some (such as the soft-skinned larvae of the Colorado potato beetle) are killed on contact.

Lepidoptera

From numerous field trials (notably on various moths), it appears that larvae of most lepidopterous pests are highly sensitive to neem. Indeed, it seems likely that armyworms, fruit borers, corn borers, and related pests will become the main targets of neem products in the near future. Neem blocks them from feeding, although this effect is usually less important than the disruption of growth it causes.

Diptera

Many species of dipterous insects-fruit fly, face fly, botfly, horn fly, and housefly, for example-are targets for neem products. Mosquitoes, too, are a possibility.

Hymenoptera

The freely feeding and caterpillar-like larvae of sawflies are target insects as well. In this group, neem's antifeedant and growth regulatory effects are both important.

Heteroptera

The "true" bugs-including many pests such as the rice bug, the green vegetable bug, and the East African coffee bug that suck juices from crops and trees-are affected by neem products. Neem's systemic qualities affect their feeding behavior and disrupt their growth and development.

Order	Insect	Action	Critical Stages of Insect
Orthoptera	Grasshoppers, crickets, Katydids	Antifeedent,	Adult
Homoptera	Cicadas, Aphids, Scale insects, leaf hoppers	Antifeedent, Growth Regulators	Larvae and Adults

Thysonoptera	Thrips	Growth Regulators	Larvae in soil, adults
Coleoptera	Beetles, Weevils	Antifeedent, Growth Retardant	Larvae
Lepidoptera	Moths, Skippers, Millers, Butterflies	Growth deterrent, antifeedent	Larvae
Diptera	Flies	Repellent	Adult
Hymenoptera	Bees, Wasps, Saw flies, ants	Antifeedent, Growth regulators	Larvae
Heteroptera	Bugs	Antifeedent, Growth deterrent	Adults

EXAMPLES

Neem's effects vary with different insects. Some effects on a small selection of major pests are summarized below.

Desert Locust

Recent laboratory research has shown that neem oil causes "solitarization" of gregarious locust nymphs. After exposure to doses equal to a mere 2.5 liters per hectare, the juveniles fail to form the massive, moving, marauding plagues that are so destructive of crops and trees. Although alive, they became solitary, lethargic, almost motionless, and thus extremely susceptible to predators such as birds. Neem affects grasshopper nymphs similarly.

This discovery differs from earlier ones on locusts. Those first approaches used alcoholic extracts and were aimed at disrupting metamorphosis or at stopping adult locusts from feeding on crops. The new approach uses neem oil enriched with azadirachtin to prevent locusts from developing into their migratory swarms. It apparently blocks the formation of the hormones and the pheromones needed to maintain the yellow-and-black gregarious form, which plagues and Africa and the Middle East. In an interesting aside, it has been shown that neem oil destroys their antennae, even when applied to the abdomen.

Neem trees grow well throughout the locust zones of Africa and the Middle East, and thus, in principle at least, the means to control the plagues could be locally produced.

Cockroach

Neem kills young cockroaches and inhibits the adults from laying eggs. Baits impregnated with a commercial preparation of neem-seed extract proved to retard the growth of oriental, brown-banded, and German cockroaches. First-instar nymphs of all three species failed to develop, and all died within 10 weeks. Last instar nymphs exhibited retarded growth, and half of them died within 9 weeks. After 24 weeks, only 2 out of the 10 surviving German-cockroach nymphs had reached adulthood.

In a "taste test," American cockroach adults preferred neem-treated pellets over untreated ones, but neem-treated milk cartons repelled them.

Brown Planthopper

Neem cake (the residue left after oil has been removed from the kernel) has proved so successful that Philippine farmers are already using it on a trial basis against the brown plant-hopper (and other rice pests). Neem oil is being employed as well. Five applications of a 25percent neem-oil emulsion sprayed with an ultra-low-volume applicator is said to protect rice crops against this increasingly severe scourge. Neem products greatly reduce the tungo virus transmission efficiency of green leaf hopper in rice.

It has been estimated that one neem tree provides enough ingredients to protect a hectare of rice. This use alone exemplifies the economic importance of further developing the neem tree for pest control.

Stored-Product Insects

Neem shows considerable potential for controlling pests of stored products. This is one of the oldest uses in Asia, and the literature contains many references to its benefits. In the traditional practice, neem leaves are mixed with grain kept in storage for 3-6 months. The ingredients responsible for keeping out the stored-grain pests are not yet identified-but they work well.

In this connection, repellency seems of primary importance. For instance, treating jute sacks with neem oil or neem extracts prevents pests-in particular, weevils (*Sitophilus species*) and flour beetles (*Tribolium species*)-from penetrating for several months. For this use, the degradation problem caused by sunlight is less of a concern because the products are mostly away from the sunlight, inside jars or other containers.

Neem oil is an extremely effective and cheap protection for stored beans, cowpeas, and other legumes. It keeps them free of bruchid-beetle infestations for at least 6 months, regardless of whether the beans were infested before treatment or not. This process may be unsuited for use in large-scale food stores, but it is potentially valuable for household use and for protecting seeds being held for planting. The treatment in no way inhibits the capacity of the seeds to germinate.

Neem has also been used in India to protect stored roots as well as tubers against the potato moth. Small amounts of neem powder are said to extend the storage life of potatoes 3 months.

Armyworm

Azadirachtin has proved an effective prophylactic against armyworms at extremely low concentrations-a mere 10 mg per hectare. For instance, it inhibits the fall armyworm, one of the most devastating pests of food crops in the western hemisphere. It has, however, been found necessary to treat the crop before the insects arrive. If this is done, they "march right on past the fields," but once they have taken up residence, it is harder to get them to move on.

Colorado Potato Beetle

In advanced trials in the United States, neem extracts have controlled the Colorado potato beetle. This is a significant pest in North America and Europe that is becoming increasingly resistant to broad-spectrum insecticides.

In experiments in Virginia, for example, neem-seed extracts (at relatively low concentrations of 0.4 per cent, 0.8 percent, and 1.2 percent) were tested in potato fields both with and without the synergist piperonyl butoxide (PBO). All treatments significantly lowered the potato beetle populations and raised potato yields; however, the extracts containing PBO were the most effective. The sprayings were most effective when the larvae were young, and were best when conducted as soon as the eggs hatched.

Leafminers

When birch trees were sprayed to control the birch leafminer (*Fenusa pusilla*), neem extract seemed to perform as well as the registered commercial pesticide Diazinon®. It was, however, slower acting, and the insects continued to damage trees before they died. This leafminer is a serious pest in parts of North America, often browning the crowns of entire forests.

The U.S. Environmental Protection Agency has approved a neem seed-extract formulation for use on leafminers. This commercial product, now available almost nationwide, is expected to be especially useful against those leafminers that attack horticultural crops. Added to the soil, neem compounds enter the roots and move up into the crop's leaves so that leafminers munching on the leaves get their molting-hormone jammed and they end up fatally trapped inside their own juvenile skins.

European Corn Borer

The European corn borer, a highly adaptable pest of com and other crops, was introduced to North America in 1917 and subsequently slashed Canada's corn yields in half. Today, it infests 40 million acres of com in the United States each year, and in just an average year American farmers spend an estimated $400 million on chemicals to fight it.

Laboratory tests using neem products on this corn borer larvae produced 100 percent mortality at 10 ppm azadirachtin; 90 per cent mortality at 1 ppm. Lower concentrations (0. 1 ppm azadirachtin) left the larvae apparently unaffected, but the adults that later emerged had grossly altered sex ratios (there were many more males than females) and the few remaining females laid fewer eggs and laid them too late. This combination of effects suggests that azadirachtin could be effective for controlling this terrible pest.

Mosquitoes

The larvae of a number of mosquito species (including Aedes and Anopheles) are sensitive to neem. They stop feeding and die within 24 hours after treatment. If neem derivatives are used alone, relatively high concentrations are required to obtain high mortality. Nonetheless, the use of simple and cheap neem products seems promising for treating pools and ponds in the towns and villages of developing countries. In one test, crushed neem seeds thrown into pools proved nearly as effective at preventing mosquito breeding as methoprene, a rather expensive pesticide that is usually imported in developing countries.

Aphids

In the Dominican Republic, water extracts of neem seed proved effective against Aphis gossypii on cucumber and okra and against *Lipaphis erysimi* on cabbage. This was in direct-contact sprays.

As noted earlier, neem extracts applied in a systemic manner (that is, within plants) usually have little effect on aphids. Apparently, this is because aphids feed only on the phloem tissues, where, for some unknown reason, neem materials accumulate least.

Fruit Files

Fruit flies (including the notorious med fly) are among the most serious horticultural pests. They cause millions of dollars in damage to fruits, and their very presence in the tropics is keeping dozens of delicious fruits from becoming major items of international trade. But, at least in experiments, the medfly is proving susceptible to neem. This insect pupates underground, and in trials in Hawaii, spraying dilute neem solution under fruit trees resulted in 100 per cent control.

More important, the neem materials were compatible with the biological-control organisms (braconid wasps) used to control fruit flies. When neem was applied to soil at levels that completely inhibited the pest from emerging from pupation, the parasites developing in these pupae emerged and exhibited normal life spans and reproductive rates. Thus, neem is compatible with biological control of fruit flies. Diazinon®, the current soil treatment for fruit flies, kills not only fruit flies but their internal parasites as well.

Gypsy Moth

The U.S. Environmental Protection Agency has approved a newsfeed-extract formulation for use on gypsy moth, a pest that is ravaging forests in parts of North America. In laboratory trials, a commercial neem formulation (Margosan-O®) produced 100 per cent kill at very low concentrations (0.2 liters per hectare). After 25 days, the larvae were shrivelled, had stopped eating, and were dying. Field tests are in progress.

Horn Flies

Ground-up neem seed and stabilized neem extracts can prevent horn flies from breeding in cattle manure. In recent U.S. Department of Agriculture trials in Kerrville, Texas, cattle were fed a diet containing these neem materials in the feed. The animals readily consumed feed containing 0.1-1 percent ground neem seed. The neem compounds passed through the digestive tract and into the manure where they kept the fly larvae from developing.

Blowflies

In Australia neem products have been tested against blowflies on sheep. The larvae of these pests penetrate and burrow under the skin of sheep. They are a major economic burden to

Australia's farmers because many of the sheep die. In the tests, azadirachtin kept blowflies from "striking" (that is, laying their eggs on sheep).

As a result of the excitement this discovery engendered, 1,000 hectares of neem have been planted in Queensland at a cost of more than $4 million. At least one Australian company has been established to produce and distribute neem products to sheep farmers. This opens up an interesting new line of neem application in animal husbandry.

NEEM ON THE MAJOR PESTS

Pest	Mode of Action
Desert Locust	Neem oil causes solitarization of gregarious nymphs at 2.5 l/ha. They became solitary, lethargic, almost motionless and highly susceptible to predators like birds
Cockroach	Neem seed extracts kills young cockroaches. Adults inhibited from laying eggs
Green Leaf Hoppers	Inhibits feeding
Brown Plant Hoppers	Reduction in survival, affect the development of nymphs to adults stage, oviposition deterrent, sterility, repellent, mating failure
Mosquito	Throwing crush neem seed in ponds prevent breeding, affect larvae
Mexican Bean Beetle	Retard growth, inhibit feeding, disrupt molting
Khapra Beetle	Inhibits feeding, disrupt molting, toxic to larvae
Bean Aphid	Reduces fecundity, disrupt molting
Diamond Back Moth	Strongly suppresses larvae and pupae, retard growth, Inhibit feeding
Pink Boll Worm	Retard growth, Inhibit feeding
Army Worm	Retard growth, Repel adult, Inhibit feeding, Disrupt molting, Toxic to larvae
Mealy Bugs	Repelles, Inhibit feeding
Rice, Cowpea and Boll Weevils	Inhibit feeding, Disrupt growth, toxic
Cabbage loopers	Inhibit feeding
Rice gall midge	Toxic

Gypsy Moth	Retard growth, Inhibit feeding, Disrupt molting
Leaf Minor	Larvae unable to molt, Retard Growth,Inhibit Feeding, Toxic
Fire ant	Inhibit feeding, Disrupt growth
Fruit flies	Repellent, (100 % control by neem spay under tree)
Nematode	Inhibit hatching, prevent second stage juvenile(neem cake)
White fly	Repellent, growth retardent, feeding inhibitor
Sorghum shoot fly	Feeding inhibitor
Spotted cucumber beetle	Growth retardent, feeding inhibitor
Snails	Kills snails

Pest Resistance to Neem Materials

A few herbivorous insects, including Homoptera, Coleoptera, and Lepidoptera do survive on neem but, largely, it is free from serious pest problems. Although Taylor indicated that insects may possibly adapt to limonoid rather quickly, but Vollinger demonstrated that two genetically different starins of *P. xylostella* treated with a neem seed extract showed no sign of resistance in feeding and fecundity tests up to 35 generations. In contrast, deltamethrin-treated lines developed resistance factor of 20 in one line and 35 in the other.

There was no cross resistance between deltamethrin and neem seed extract in the deltamethrin-resistant lines. Also, the esterase and multi-function oxidase enzyme activity did not change during the 35 generations. The diversity of neem allelochemicals and their combined behavioural and physiological effects on insect pests seem to confer a built-in resistance prevention mechanism in neem. However, wisdom demands that users should refrain from exclusive and extended application of single bioactive materials, such as azadirachtin.

Effects on Other Organisms

Although neem's effects on pestiferous insects are by far the best known, the tree's various products can influence other pest organisms as well. In the long run, these may well prove the most important of all. At present, however, the effects on non-insect pests are poorly understood. This chapter highlights some of the findings to date.

NEMATODES

Neem products affect various types of nematodes. This may be significant because certain of these thread worms are among the most devastating agricultural pests and are also among the most difficult to control. In addition, an increasing number of synthetic nematocides have had to be withdrawn from the market for toxicological reasons.

Today, there is a small but increasing body of evidence that neem might provide useful replacements. Certain limonoid fractions extracted from neem kernels are proving active against root-knot nematodes, the type most devastating to plants. They inhibit the larvae from emerging and the eggs from hatching, and in at least one test they have done so at concentrations in the parts-per-million range. Water extracts of neem cake (the residue remaining after the oil has been pressed out of the seeds) are also nematocidal.

In a careful trial in Aligarh, India, amending soil with sawdust and neem cake dropped the root-knot index to zero and, of all the treatments tested, gave the greatest growth of tomatoes, a crop that is very sensitive to these nematodes.

In tests in a greenhouse and in the field in Germany, tomato plants were obviously improved by neem products, but there was no significant difference in the numbers of some nematode species in the soil. However, among treated and untreated soils the majority was extracted from the roots of plants in untreated soil.

Cardamom growers in South India are already using neem cake to control nematodes. Of 19 growers interviewed recently, 17 said that nothing works as well. These were sophisticated farmers who monitor world cardamom prices regularly and use synthetic chemicals for controlling other pests in their fields. In other words, they weren't using neem out of ignorance or poverty. They incorporate 100-259 kg per hectare of neem cake in their cardamom fields every year. About 3000 tons of neem cake are now used annually in India's Cardamom Hills. It is sold by pesticide dealers, who transport it from 250-300 km away.

SNAILS

Various neem extracts kill snails. This appears to be beneficial in some cases. In laboratory tests, for example, ethanol extracts proved toxic to the aquatic snail (*Biamphalaria glabrata*), a species that is necessary to the life cycle of the parasite causing schistosomiasis (bilharzia). The extracts killed both the adult snail and its eggs. This raises the possibility that neem products may find a role in controlling schistosomiasis, a horrible scourge that infects some 200 million people in the tropics.

In another test, an aqueous solution of neem fruit resulted in a 100 percent kill of *Melania scabra*. This snail, common throughout the Orient, is a vector of lung flukes, a parasitic flatworm that encysts in the lungs of livestock, wildlife, and people, causing debilitation and sometimes death.

CRUSTACEANS

Little is known about neem's effects -beneficial or detrimental- on crustaceans. However, in one intriguing set of experiments in the Philippines, it proved beneficial.

In rice paddies, the ostracod *Heterocypris luzonensis* feeds on the blue-green algae that fix nitrogen from the air. This minute aquatic crustacean thereby reduces a source of fertilizer for the crop. Killing this tiny creature thus would indirectly boost the nitrogen available and probably increase rice yields. Aqueous neem-kernal extracts have killed it very effectively under laboratory conditions.

FUNGI

Neem has demonstrated antifungal activity. Should this prove widely applicable, the availability of a natural fungicide that can be grown, extracted, and applied by farmers themselves could be of great consequence to worldwide agriculture and food supply. Fungi attack crops in countless numbers and forms. They are constantly evolving enemies of farms and forests. Many can reach epidemic proportions, a few have no cures, and some can make certain crops impossible to grow. And, despite the best of modern science, they still threaten wheat, com, rice, and other plants that feed the world.

Not a lot is known about neem's practical use against rots, smuts, wilts, mildews, die-backs, and other fungal plant diseases. However, several tests have indicated considerable promise.

In one test, neem oil protected the seeds of chickpeas against the serious fungal diseases *Rhizocionia solani*, *Sclerotium rolfsii*, and *Sclerotinia sclerotiorum*. It also slowed the growth of *Fusarium oxysporum* but did not kill it. In addition, neem cake incorporated into the soil completely blocked the development of the resting forms of *R. solani*- thereby interfering with the long-term survival of this devastating fungus.

In another, neem-seed extracts showed beneficial effects against leaf fungi. Spraying crude neem oil on lilac bushes, when done before any sign of outbreak, prevented powdery mildew from breaking out for the rest of the season. This protectant also gave essentially 100 percent control on hydrangeas in greenhouses-better than Beniate® (benomyl), the standard mildew treatment in much of the world.

In the case of bean rust, neem extracts have given 90 percent control when applied before the plants were exposed to the fungus. However, they worked poorly once rust was established.

In addition to affecting root-knot nematodes, treating soil with neem can reduce the populations of pest fungi in the rhizosphere that attack and feed off plant roots.

Aflatoxin

A truly unusual and potentially notable connection between neem and fungi has recently been reported from Louisiana. In trials there, neem-leaf extract failed to kill the fungus *Aspergillus flavus*, but, against all expectations, it completely stopped it from producing aflatoxin.

Greenhouse studies have since confirmed these laboratory findings. The extracts appear to halt the formation of substances called polyketides, which the fungi convert into aflatoxin. The enzymes for the conversion remain in place, but key chemicals they need to synthesize the feared toxin are no longer available.

It proved easy to take advantage of this in practice: neem leaves were mashed in water, the liquid separated, and it was applied without further refinement. This crude liquid extract turned off aflatoxin production in both laboratory cultures and cotton bolls on living plants.

These findings could be of immense significance. Aflatoxin causes liver cancer, and under hot and humid conditions, where fungi thrive, it can form on peanuts, corn, cottonseed, and other widely eaten food crops. It is of great concern these days; it not only threatens health, it also promises economic catastrophe. For example, the United States may soon be banned from exporting cottonseed to feed Europe's cattle. The U.S. aflatoxin limit is 20 pass per billion (ppb), but Europe's goal for the future is a mere 2 ppb in feed and only 0.5 ppb in milk. Also, aflatoxin-contaminated local foods and feeds are causing increased concern in Asia and Africa.

PLANT VIRUSES

Plant viruses pose some of the most severe threats to world agriculture. Because they invade the crop's cells and cloak themselves with the plant's normal life processes, they are far more difficult to control than free-living organisms such as bacteria, protozoa, or fungi. At present, we can only try to halt their spread-something nearly impossible to achieve under even the best of circumstances-because viruses "hitch rides" in insects such as aphids, as well as on dirty tools, blowing dust, or spreading floodwaters.

A few virus-inhibiting chemicals are known for treating human and animal diseases (AZT for AIDS, for instance), but at present, none are available for treating plants. Neem might be the first. Crude extracts seem to bind certain plant viruses effectively, and so limit infection.

However, for the moment at least, neem seems most effective at interfering with the transmission of plant viruses carried by insects. This conclusion is drawn from several successful tests of neem's effects against insect vectors of plant viruses.

These tests include the following:

- A trial in the Philippines where rice fields sprayed with neem oil had significantly lower incidence of the ragged-stunt virus, which affects rice and is transmitted by the brown planthopper.
- A second trial in the Philippines where mixtures of neem oil and custard-apple oil interfered with the transmission of tungro virus, another rice pest.
- Experiments in India where neem-leaf extracts reduced the transmission of tobacco mosaic, a virus that seriously affects several vegetable crops.
- Field trials in the Philippines where fields treated with urea and neem cake were found to be lower in viral diseases than those treated with urea alone.
- Enzyme-linked immunosorbent assays showing that rice seedlings grown in soil treated with neem cake were significantly freer of rice tungro viruses (transmitted by green rice leafhopper) than those in untreated control plots.

On the other hand, not all trials have been this successful. In the United States, daily applications of neem leaf extracts over a month's time to turnip plants infected with cauliflower mosaic virus did not reduce viral infection.

NONTARGET SPECIMENS

Neem extracts proved to be "soft" on unintended targets. Further examples follow.

Earthworms

In greenhouse studies, when neem leaves and seed kernels were incorporated into potting soil containing earthworms (*Eisenia foetida*), the number of young worms produced increased 25 percent. In field trials there were no differences in the number of worms, but the average weight of each worm was highest in neem-treated plots. Thus, it seems possible that neem products can favor earthworms, at least under certain conditions.

Beneficial Insects

Neem seems remarkably benign to spiders, butterflies, and insects such as bees that pollinate crops and trees, ladybugs that consume aphids, and wasps that act as parasites on various crop pests. In the main, this is because neem products must be ingested to be effective. Thus, insects that feed on plant tissues succumb, while those that feed on nectar or other insects rarely contact significant concentrations of neem products.

All this is coming clearer from recent research. For example, only after repeated spraying of highly concentrated neem products onto plants in flower were worker bees at all affected. Under these extreme conditions, the workers carried contaminated pollen or nectar to the hives and fed it to the brood. Small hives then showed insect-growth-regulating effects; however, medium-sized and large bee populations were unaffected.

Under laboratory conditions the larvae of ladybugs and lacewings have shown some insect-growth-regulating effects from neem picked up from the bodies of other insects. However, in greenhouse trials in Florida, neem products proved essentially nontoxic to predators and parasitoids of the cotton aphid and the sweet potato whitefly. Neither the amount of predation nor of parasitism was notably reduced.

A census of natural aphid enemies collected from seven different field trials indicated that neem has no detrimental effects on either predators (coccinellids, chrysopids, syrphids) or parasitoids (ichneurnonids, braconids). The aphids in the neem-treated plots were actually carrying more parasites than were those in either the control plots or the plots treated with the insecticide pyrethrum.

Chapter **15**

Neem Extracts

Neem is attracting worldwide attention in recent decades mainly due to its bioactive ingredients that find increasing use in modern crop and grain protection. Described here are some easy methods by which the neem extracts can be prepared by the farmer himself:

The whole neem tree contains bitters in varied extent, but higher concentration of it is found in the neem kernel. Neem kernel is a valuable source of major limnoids responsible for pest contol. Hence good qulity of neem fruit is essential for production of high quality neem extract. It is therefore essential to understand the scientific method of fruit colletion and depulping.

METHODS OF PREPARATION

NEEM FRUIT COLLECTION AND DEPULPING

Neem Fruit Collection

The neem yields fruits during May to August every year. The ripend fruits to be collected for the processing. Cover the ground below neem tree with cotton or jute cloth, or shade net to avoid contact of neem fuits with soil. It will also facilitate the collection of the fruits. Being rich in carbohydrates neem fruits gets attacked by fungi when came in contact with soil. Such fruits may get infected with toxin developing fungus and may damage the qulity of the final products prepared from these fuits. Hence it is strongly recommended to avoid contact of neem fruits with soil. As the fruit ripes during rainy season they must depulped as early as possible. Avoid storage of fresh, wet fuits in the plastic bags. Use bamboo baskets or jute bags for storage.

Depulping of Neem Fruits

Depulping is a process to remove seed coat and pulp form the neem seed. It is done by hand and using mechanical depulper. Rub the ripe neem fruits between palms in the bucket of water and wash the seed. Use clean water for depulping. Neem Research and Technology Development Centre (NRTDC) developed a mechnical depulper to handle large quantity of neem fruits. After depulping and cleaning dry the neem seed in the shade in a thin layer. Select the place with good airation.Do not make heap of the seed. Protect it from direct rains. After drying neem seed upto 11% moisture store it in a jute gunny bags or bamboo baskets. Do not store in plastic bags as it may damage the quality of seed. Keep the neem seed in a cool and dry place. If processed properly these neem seeds can be stroed for 6-12 months. It is recommended to use neem seed for prepariton of extract or oil extraction after 3 months and before 8 months. The highest concentration of limnoids and oil found after 3 month and before 8 months period.

Neem Kernel Aqueous Extract:

The simple method of Neem Kernel Aqueous Extract preparation consist of following steps -

Take dried neem seed. Decorticate (Removal of seed coat) it with the help of mortar and pastle or any mechnical decorticator. Clean the neem kernel and seed coat mixture by winnowing seed coat.

Weigh 1 kg of clean neem kernel and make powder of grain size like fine tea powder. It should be pounded in such a way that no oil comes out. Soak it in a about 10 lits of clean water. Add 10 ml of pH neutal adjuvant (mixture of emulsifier, spreader etc.) and stir the mixture. Keep the mixture overnight and filter it on the next day with clean muslin cloth. Put water in the residue and repeat the extraction 2-3 times. Use residue as a manure for plants.

Spraying of NKAE

The spraying of 1.25% to 5% (Neem Kernel wt. Basis) of NKAE is recommended on the crops. The use of is recommended as a preventive at lower concentrartion and protective at higher concentaton i.e. uptp 5 %. Use the spray solution on the same day. Spraying should be done in the low intensity of sunlight preferablery in the afternoon. The effect of the NKAE remains for 7-10 days. Care to be taken to cover all plant foliage with NKAE.

Neem Leaf Extract:

For 5 litres of water, 1 kg of green neem leaf is required. Since the quantity of leaves required for preparation of this extract is quite high (nearly 80 kg are required for 1 hectare) this can be used for nursery and kitchen gardens. The leaves are soaked overnight in water. The next day the leaves are grounds and the extract is filtered. The extract is beneficial against leaf eating caterpillars, grubs, locusts and grasshoppers. To the extract, emulsifier is added as mentioned in kernel extract.

Neem Cake Extract:

100 gms of Neem cake is required for 1 litre of water. The Neem cake is put in a muslin pouch and soaked in water. It is soaked overnight before use in the morning. It is then filtered and emulsifier is added -1-ml for 1-litre of water. It can then be used for spraying.

Neem Oil Spray:

15-30 ml Neem oil is added to 1 litre of water and stirred well. To this emulsifier is added (1ml/1litre). It is very essential to add the emulsifier and mix properly. This should be used immediately before the oil droplets start floating. A knapsack sprayer is better for Neem oil spraying in preference to a hand sprayer.

Precatutions for using Neem Extracts/Formulations :

Spraying should be undertaken in the morning or late in the afternoon. Insects lay eggs on the underside of the leaves. Hence it is important to spray on the underside of the leaves as well.

Caution

The active principles of Neem are destroyed by

- Heating and boiling the extract- do not boil the mixture,
- Acidic or alkaline pH emulsifier- use neutral pH emulsifier,
- Ultraviole rays of sulight - Spray during moderate sulight,
- Hydrolysis of water- use aquous extract on same day.

Chapter 16

Neem Oil

Neem oil is a botanical pesticide made from an extract of the plant *Azadirachta indica*. Since it doesn't strongly affect humans, mammals, or beneficial bugs, farmers use neem oil as an insecticide and miticide to keep away pests like aphids and white flies. Neem oil even protects crops from fungal infections such as mildew and rust. People use insecticide with neem oil to repel mosquitoes and lice.

The plant that gives us neem oil originates in Southeast Asia. People from these countries have long noted the benefits of crushing the leaves and stems against their skin to keep off biting insects like gnats.

A wider industrial and commercial use was found for the potent oil by grinding the seeds of the neem plant. The neem seed kernel is very rich in fatty acids, often up to 50 percent of the kernel's weight. Neem seed oil is very bitter with a garlic/sulfur smell and contains vitamin E and other essential amino acids.

Studies of the various components of the oil have found the percentages of the following fatty acids:

- oleic acid - 52.8%
- stearic acid - 21.4%
- palmitic acid - 12.6%
- linoleic acid - 2.1%
- various lower fatty acids - 2.3%

The percentages vary from sample to sample depending on place and time of collection of the seeds. When the oil is distilled from seeds, its concentrated mixture contains high amounts of the active chemical azadirachtin.

Azadirachtin-rich neem oil gets sprayed on crops as an organic substitute for other harsher insecticides that might be carcinogenic or have limited uses. Neem oil repels harmful insects like white flies, gnats, aphids, mites, and weevils, as well as strengthening the crops against rust, scab, mildew, and blight. Edible crops of vegetables do not get poisoned when neem oil is used.

Neem oil makes the plants it touches taste bitter, so pests won't eat them, as a "contact" insecticide. Azadirachtin also interrupts insects' transitions between different stages of metamorphosis, such as growing from larvae to pupae. It prevents insects from developing a hardened exoskeleton. When the chemical gets absorbed through the roots of crops, it functions as a "systemic insecticide." That means crops don't need to be constantly re-sprayed.

The greatest benefit of using neem oil is that it doesn't harm beneficial insects. Butterflies, earthworms, and bees all help plants pollinate or absorb nutrients. Lacewings eat insects trying to feed on the crops. But these bugs won't have a negative reaction to neem oil or azadirachtin.

Neem oil is excellent moisturizing oil that contains compounds with historical and scientific validity as medicinals. Neem oil has even made it into cosmetic and household products. Use of the oil for cosmetics and medicines has been limited by its strongly bitter taste and sulfur/garlic smell. Only when it was made into soaps or strong chemical alternatives was it acceptable use by most people. Lotions and skin sprays use the oil as a mild insecticide that isn't likely to cause rashes. If you soak cotton balls in neem oil and place them in your closet, it will dissuade wool moths from devouring your clothes. It is no wonder the leaves have been substituted for the oil to get the benefits of neem.

Obtaining quality neem oil

To bring the many therapeutic effects of neem oil to all the people that could benefit from them requires a major change in neem oil's quality. From the picking of the fruit to filling the oil into drums, careful attention to quality is the only way to get the best oil possible. It is now known that if the neem seed is not dried and stored properly and the oil is not expressed in a hygienic way the oil will be very dark, have a foul odour and may contain dangerous contaminants.

Methods for obtaining neem oil:

The first thing to consider is the collection of the seeds. Neem is not considered a plantation tree in India so the seeds must be gathered from wild trees growing on the fringes of farms, along hillsides and from roadsides and shade trees around homes in the rural villages. Collection of the seeds is a seasonal affair that has historically been organized by cooperatives that press the oil from the seeds for soap manufacture.

As the ripe fruit falls to the ground, it is gathered from around the trees. Some of the fruit will have been eaten by birds and the seeds excreted. Other fruit may have been on the ground for weeks, covered with mold or simply rotten. The collected fruit is then carried to a water supply to wash away the fruit covering the seed. After washing, the seeds are set out to dry in the sun. The dry seeds are bagged and sold to village merchants who later sell them to an oil processing facility.

There are three main processes for extracting the oil from the seed kernels with some companies using combinations. The one used since antiquity is the mechanical press method. Neem seed kernels are place into a tub and either a screw or some form of press is used to squeeze the kernels under pressure until the oil is pressed out and collected.

The second method uses steam and high pressures to extract the oil. The kernels are heated with steam to increase the oil flow then squeezed under high pressure. Most of the oil is extracted from the kernels but it is dark and smelly with many of the active compounds destroyed by the high temperatures.

The third and newest method is solvent extraction. This method is used by most seed oil processors since almost all of the oil is removed from the kernels. The neem seed kernels are finely ground and placed into a container along with a petroleum solvent, usually hexane (white gasoline). The neem oil is captured by the solvent and is pulled out of the kernels. The solvent/neem oil mixture is then put into a vat where most of the solvent is recovered leaving the neem oil and minute traces of the solvent behind. Sometimes seed cake obtained after mechanical pressing is further extracted using this method. Many of neem oil's active compounds are not soluble in hexane and are left behind in the solvent extraction process.

Once the oil has been extracted, it is usually put into metal drums for storage and shipment. Since neem oil is used primarily for soap manufacture by small manufacturers, there has been no demand for pure or clean neem oil. Therefore, inexpensive second-hand drums are used to store the oil. With used drums, there is the possibility of contaminating the neem oil with dangerous chemicals that could have been previously stored in the drums. Purchasing neem oil in the open marketplace will usually provide the purchaser with very low quality oil that is potentially contaminated.

The best method for obtaining quality neem oil with a majority of the active compounds intact is cold pressed. In cold pressing the oil is lighter in colour with milder odour. There is also the elimination of any potential residual solvents in the oil that could pose health hazards to the consumer. The downside is that high quality cold pressed neem oil is more expensive to produce than solvent extracted oil and is much harder to obtain. Few processors are willing to forego the loss of any of the oil that could have been extracted by solvent and have quit using cold presses.

Improved method for obtaining neem oil:

Experiments with the collection, storage and extraction procedures have disclosed that the main reason the oil was typically bad was the very procedures traditionally used. The seeds were often old and rancid before they were even collected. Storing the seeds in the hot, humid Indian summer made them even worse. By the time they were processed, the kernels were black and smelly which resulted in black, smelly oil.

A better method requires the collection of seeds specifically for the manufacture of quality health and beauty aid products. Light green kernels from fresh seeds yield a light oil with only a slight odour and a tolerable bitter taste. To get this high-quality oil, neem fruit has to be picked from the trees rather than gathered off the ground.

The fresh fruit then has to be taken to a facility where it is washed to remove the fruit from the seeds and the clean seeds quickly air dried. Dried seeds are then de-husked and the kernels cold pressed. The kernels should only be pressed once to obtain "virgin" oil, guaranteeing only the oil is removed leaving the waxy and tar-like substances behind. The light neem oil must then be stored in new drums for shipment to the manufacturing facility. This method produces high-quality neem oil suitable for use in any health and beauty aid product.

Chapter 17

Azadirachtin

TRADE OR OTHER NAMES

Modern Science has isolated & identified AZADIRACHTIN as the chief active ingredient in Neem responsible for the insect-pest growth regulators.

Empirical formula	:	C 35 H 44 O 16
Molecular weight	:	720
Chemical family	:	Tetranortriterpenoids
Trade names	:	Align, Azatin and Turplex. Formulations include a 10% plant extract (technical) and a 3% EC.
Sources	:	Neem fruit seed kernel

INTRODUCTION

The key insecticidal ingredient found in the neem tree is azadirachtin, a naturally occurring substance that belongs to an organic molecule class called tetranortriterpenoids. It is structurally similar to insect hormones called "ecdysones," which control the process of metamorphosis as the insects pass from larva to pupa to adult. Metamorphosis requires the careful synchrony of many hormones and other physiological changes to be successful, and azadirachtin seems to be an "ecdysone blocker." It blocks the insect's production and release of these vital hormones. Insects then will not molt, thus breaking their life cycle. Azadirachtin may also serve as a feeding deterrent for some insects. Depending on the stage of life-cycle, insect death may not occur for several days. However, upon ingestion of minute quantities, insects become quiescent and stop feeding.

Residual insecticidal activity is evident for 7 to 10 days or longer, depending on insect and application rate. Azadirachtin is used to control whiteflies, aphids, thrips, fungus gnats, caterpillars, beetles, mushroom flies, mealy bugs, leaf miners, gypsy moths and others on food, greenhouse crops, ornamentals and turf.

AZADIRACHTIN ACTS IN THE FOLLOWING WAY:

- Disturbing or inhibiting the development of the eggs, larvae, or pupae.
- Blocking the moulting of larvae or nymphs.
- Disturbing mating and sexual communication.
- Repelling larvae and adults.
- Deterring females from laying eggs.
- Sterilising adults.
- Deterring feeding.

Advantages:

1. Broad spectrum of activity.
2. No known insecticide resistance mechanisms.
3. Compatible with many commercial insecticides and fungicides.
4. New mode of action with possible multiple sites of attack.
5. Classified as a biological insecticide for registration purposes.
6. Low use rates.
7. Compatible with other biological agents for IPM Programme.
8. Not persistent in the environment.
9. Minimal impact of Non-target organisms.
10. Formulation flexibility.
11. No re-entry restrictions.
12. Supply available from pre-existing infrastructure.
13. Application flexibility - can be sprayed or drenched.
14. Non-phototoxic formulations available.

TOXICOLOGICAL EFFECTS

ACUTE TOXICITY

The acute oral toxicity in rats fed technical grade azadirachtin ranged from greater than 3,540 mg/kg to greater than 5,000 mg/kg, the highest dose tested when administered undiluted to albino rats.

The single-dose oral toxicity LD50 of the formulated product Azatin-EC fed to rats was 4,241 mg/kg; considered practically non-toxic.

The acute inhalation toxicity study in rats exposed to technical azadirachtin showed that the acute inhalation LD50 is greater than 2.41 mg/L per animal, the highest dose tested. Although this figure is below the 5.0 mg/L limit test dose for an acute inhalation study, the reported concentration was the maximum dose possible under the test conditions. No deaths occurred during the course of the study. Azadirachtin was given a toxicity classification of Category III.

The 4-hour acute inhalation LC50 in rats exposed to the formulated product Azatin-EC was >2.18 mg/kg.

A primary eye irritation study in rabbits exposed to technical azadirachtin was rated mild to moderately irritating after instillation of 0.1 gm of the undiluted material. At one hour post-instillation, the maximum eye irritation score was 15.3/110; by 24, 48, and 72 hours the scores were 6.2/110, 0.3/110, and 0/110, respectively. It was given a toxicity category of III.

Primary dermal irritation in rabbits when tested at a single dose (0.5 gm) by applying it to the shaved backs of rabbits, did not cause any dermal irritation after 4 hours of exposure. The dermal score was zero for all treated rabbits at all examination times. A toxicity category of IV, mild to slightly irritating, was assigned.

An acute dermal toxicity study of rabbits exposed to technical azadirachtin was performed. The material was applied for 24 hours at a single dose of 2.0 gm/kg to the shaved backs of the rabbits, that caused dermal irritation which resolved by day nine. Azadirachtin was classified as a mild irritant. Another study reported the dermal LD50 for rabbits to be >2,000 mg/kg.

Dermal sensitization in guinea pigs found the technical end-use product to be categorized as a mild sensitizer when administered undiluted to albino guinea pigs. The test material was considered a weak dermal sensitizer to albino guinea pigs.

CHRONIC TOXICITY

A 90-day oral toxicity study in rats fed levels of 500, 2500, and 10,000 ppm of azadirachtin showed no signs of overt systemic toxicity at any dose level after 90 days of feeding. Mean body weight was significantly decreased in the 10,000 ppm males and females at weeks 3 and 4, respectively. This persisted for the duration of the 90-day feeding period.

Reproductive Effects

Male antifertility activity of neem leaf extract was studied in mice, rats, rabbits and guinea pigs by daily oral feeding of a cold-water extract of fresh green neem leaves. The infertility effect was seen in treated male rats as there was a 66.7% reduction in fertility after 6 weeks, 80% after 9 weeks, and 100% after 11 weeks. There was no inhibition of spermatogenesis. During this period there was no decrease in body weight and no other manifestation of toxicity observed. There was a marked decrease in the mortality of spermatozoa. The infertility in rats was not associated with loss of libido or with impotence and the animals maintained normal mating behaviour. The male antifertility activity was reversible in 4 to 6 weeks. Neem extract also shows reversible male antifertility activity in mice without inhibition of spermatogenesis. In guinea pigs and rabbits, however, it exhibited toxicity as demonstrated by 66.6% and 74.9% mortality in guinea pigs and 80 and 90% mortality in rabbits at the end of 4 and 6 weeks, respectively.

Teratogenic Effects

No information was found.

Mutagenic Effects

Technical azadirachtin was evaluated for the potential to cause gene mutations in the S. typhimurium strains at any dose (5, 50, 500, 5,000 micrograms/plate) with or without S-9 activation. The study was negative.

The Ames test was negative with or without metabolic activation for the formulated product Azatin-EC. The UDS and Mouse Lymphoma studies were also negative.

Carcinogenic Effects

No information was found.

Organ Toxicity

Rats dosed with 600 mg/kg/day of the formulated product Azatin-EC for 90 days showed no overt adverse effects on target organs.

Fate in Humans and Animals

No information was found.

ECOLOGICAL EFFECTS

Effects on Birds

No significant effects on other wildlife were reported.

Effects on Aquatic Organisms

The formulated product Azatin-EC is not expected to kill fish at recommended rates. The LC50 for rainbow trout exposed to azadirachtin is 0.48 ppm. It may cause significant fish kill if large concentrations reach waterways. It breaks down rapidly (in 50-100 hours) in water or light, and is not likely to accumulate or cause long-term effects.

Effects on Other Animals (Non-target species)

Azadirachtin is relatively harmless to spiders, butterflies, and insects such as bees that pollinate crops and trees, ladybugs that consume aphids, and wasps that act as parasites on various crop pests. This is because neem products must be ingested to be effective. Thus, insects that feed on plant tissue succumb, while those that feed on nectar or other insects rarely contact significant concentrations of neem products.

Another study found that only after repeated spraying of highly concentrated neem products onto plants in flower were worker bees at all affected. Under these extreme conditions, the workers carried contaminated pollen or nectar to the hives and fed it to the brood. Small hives then showed insect-growth-regulating effects; however, medium-sized and large bee populations were unaffected.

A study of neem products and their effect on mortality, growth and reproduction of earthworms in soils was conducted. Positive effects on weight and survival were found in soil treated with ground neem leaves and ground seed kernals under greenhouse conditions. Reproduction was slightly favoured over a period of 13 weeks in a neem-enriched substrate in rearing cages. Various neem products were incorporated in the upper 10-cm soil layer of tomato plots. None of the materials had negative side effects on seven species of earthworms.

No significant effects on other wildlife were reported.

ENVIRONMENTAL FATE

Breakdown of Chemical in Soil and Groundwater

Potential for mobility in soil is very low for the formulated product Azatin-EC. Accumulation in the environment is not expected.

Breakdown of Chemical in Surface Water

The formulated product Azatin-EC which contains the active ingredient azadirachtin is considered a water pollutant. It breaks down rapidly (in 100 hours) in water or light, and will not cause long-term effects.

Breakdown of Chemical in Vegetation

Azadirachtin is considered non-phytotoxic when used as directed.

PROPERTIES AND GUIDELINES

Azadirachtin is a tetranortriterpenoid botanical insecticide of the liminoid class extracted from the neem tree *Azadirachta indica*. It is a yellow-green powder, with a strong garlic-sulphur odour. Hazardous combustion products include carbon monoxide and carbon dioxide.

Physico-chemical Properties:

Chemical name	:	Azadirachtin A, Azadirachtin B
Chemical Class/Use	:	Tetranortriterpenoid/Insect growth regulator
Specific gravity	:	1.066 (Azatin-EC)
Solubility in water	:	0.00005
Boiling point	:	25.5-100 degrees C (Margosan-O)
Flashpoint	:	>60 degrees C; >62.7 C (Azatin-EC); 13.1 degrees C (Margosan-O)
Vapor pressure	:	>2 mmHg @ 25 degrees C (Azatin-EC); 44mm @ 20 degrees C (Margosan-O)
Kow	:	12.3; partitioning from water to oil is relatively high (Azatin-EC)
Molecular Weight	:	720 (Aza A), 662 (Aza B)
Empirical Formulae	:	C35H44O16(Aza A), $C_{33}H_{42}O_{14}$(Aza B)
Physical State	:	Yellowish solid powder
Melting Point	:	160-180ºC
Storage	:	Below 20ºC
Bulk Density	:	Before Compaction -0.28, After Compaction -0.40
pH	:	6.2 + 0.02
Flash Point	:	Greater than 100ºC

Chapter 18

Fertilizers Uses

Indian farmers have traditionally used deoiled neem cake as a fertilizer in their fields. The dual activity of neem cake as fertilizer and pest repellent has made it a favoured input. Neem leaves have also been used to enrich the soil. Together, they are widely used in India to fertilize cash crops. When neem cake is ploughed into the soil it also protects plant roots from nematodes and white ants. Farmers in southern parts of India puddle neem leaves into flooded rice fields before the rice seedlings are transplanted.

ANALYSIS OF 100 kg OF NEEM SEED CAKE

Contents	Amt in Kgs
Nitrogen	3.56
Phosphorous	0.83
Potassium	1.67
Calcium	0.77
Magnesium	0.75

Application to the neem seed cake to crops provides them with various nutrients. Besides the neem seed cake also reduces the number of soil insect pests, fungi, bacteria and nematodes and protects the crop from damage caused by these organisms. Neem seed cake can also reduce alkalinity in the soil by producing organic acids when mixed with the soil. The calcium and magnesium present in neem cake also aid in removing alkalinity.

For cash crops such as tumeric, sugarcane, banana and cardamom, 200 kg per hectare of neem cake is applied. For black pepper and betelvine 250 g per plant is applied. Neem cake is also extensively used for citrus trees, jasmine, roses and vegetable crops as an organic manure.

Neem for Soil Fertility & Fertilizer Management.

Indian farmers have traditionally used deoiled neem cake as a fertilizer in their fields. The dual activity of neem cake as fertilizer and pest repellent, has made it a favored input. Neem leaves have also been used to enrich the soil. Together, they are widely used in India to fertilize cash crops. When neem cake is ploughed into the soil it also protects plant roots from nematodes and white ants.

Nutrient contents of Neem Seed Cake

CONTENTS	PER CENT
Nitrogen	3.56
Phosphorous	0.83
Potassium	1.67
Calcium	0.77
Magnesium	0.75

Application to the neem seed cake to crops provides them with various nutrients. Besides the neem seed cake also reduces the number of soil insect pests, fungi, bacteria and nematodes and protects the crop from damage caused by these organisms. Neem seed cake can also reduce alkalinity in the soil by producing organic acids when mixed with the soil.

For cash crops such as tumeric, sugarcane, banana and cardamom, 200 kg per hectare of Neem cake is applied. For black pepper and betelvine 250 g per plant is applied. Neem cake is also extensively used for citrus trees, jasmine, roses and vegetable crops as an organic manure.

Good soil fertility means good crop yields. Preventing the loss of plant nutrients from an ecosystem is important for soil-fertility management. Nitrogen, phosphorus, and potassium (N, P, K) are the three major elements which determine soil fertility and should be ideally present in 4:2:1 ratio; aberrations affect fertility and therefore crop yield. Urea, containing 46% of N, is applied to crops in the largest amounts; but less than half of this N, in the form of nitrate, is available to the crops. The rest is lost through 'leaching' or by 'volatilization', or by surface run-off after a heavy shower. Leaching of soluble nitrates into the subsoil and, eventually into ground water is well known. Nitrate losses of 50 to 70% through leaching were observed in rice crops in India.

Leaching not only depletes precious nitrate but also takes away clay, soil, and organic matter, leading to low chemical soil fertility and low plant-available water reserves. Ammonia volatilization also can contribute to a nearly 60% nitrate loss. Loss through volatilization occurs when the denitrifying bacteria reduce the nitrate to elemental nitrogen and nitrous oxide which escape to the stratosphere and cause ozone depletion and also contribute to greenhouse warming. On the other hand, nitrate build-up in drinking water can reduce the blood's ability to transport oxygen, especially if the nitrates are converted into nitrites (blue-baby syndrome). Even ruminants are vulnerable to nitrate or nitrite poisoning, leading to poor growth rates, reduced milk production, and increased susceptibility to infections, and even abortions.

One way to minimise nitrate loss is to apply the urea more than once in smaller quantities or, alternatively, to use a slow-release urea which makes the urea available in the soil for a longer time. Bains *et al.* (1971) in field trials in India found that an acetone extract of neem kernel was an excellent nitrification inhibitor, even better than sulphur-coated urea. Ammonia volatilization, urea hydrolysis, and leaching, were all reduced when urea was blended or coated with neem cake.

Results from several field experiments show that neem cake coating of prilled urea increased nitrogen uptake by 4.5 to 19.4%. The increase in rice yield due to neem cake coating/blending of prilled urea ranged from 1 to 54%, the average being 9.6%. Neem cake coated urea applied to rice or sugarcane also left a carryover effect and increased sugarcane yield by 7% in the ratoon sugarcane crop.

Ready-to-use, neem-based urea-coating agents, such as 'Nimin' (containing ca. 5% neem bitter tetranortriterpenoids) are now commercially available in India. Application of Nimin-coated urea (1 part Nimin: 100 parts urea, wt/wt) reduced losses of fertiliser N through leaching and denitrification by 30-35% and increased yields in treated crops by up to 25%. The bitters in Nimin delay the denitrification process up to 30 days by either killing nitrifying bacteria or suppressing their activity. Coating urea with Nimin could bring a saving of up to 20% of urea. The technology is becoming popular with farmers in India where annual Nimin sales are now ca. 700 metric tons.

Neem for Sustainable Agriculture and Environmental Conservation

In the past two decades, "green revolution technologies" have more than doubled the yield potential of rice and wheat, especially in Asia. These high-input production systems requiring massive quantities of fertilisers, pesticides, irrigation, and machines, however, disregard the ecological integrity of land, forests, and water resources, endanger the flora and fauna, and cannot be sustained over generations. Also, we cannot look to the sea in future as fishing stocks in many parts of the world are already in crisis due to overfishing or pollution. To a great extent, future food security and economic independence of developing countries would depend on improving the productivity of biophysical resources through the application of sustainable production methods, by improving tolerance of crops to adverse environmental conditions, and by reducing crop and post-harvest losses caused by pests and diseases.

Environmentally Friendly Agricultural Technologies

Appropriate technologies, which do not assault the nature, would have key roles to play in ensuring food security, in improving human health, and in rehabilitating and conserving the environment to safeguard the well being of the posterity. Instead of striving for more "green revolutions" with emphasis on miracle seeds, hard-hitting, synthetic and engineered pesticides, and increased use of fertilizers, the future must look to natural ways and processes for augmenting agricultural productivity.

In fact, all development efforts and activities should be within well defined ecological rules rather than within narrow economic gains. Sustainable agricultural systems must be ecologically sound for long-term food sufficiency, equitable in providing social justice, and ethical in respecting both future generations and other species. For developing countries, the use of the neem tree may provide a key component in more sustainable agricultural system including pest and nutrient management, human health, and environmental conservation.

Chapter 19

A Blessing to the Environment

NEEM AND ENVIRONMENT

Neem has powerful pest controlling activities and medicinal properties. More importantly, pesticides made from neem are much safer compared to synthetic pesticides. The side-effects of the synthetic pesticides are often not less serious than the problems themselves. They cause environmental contamination and are a great risk of human health. As a consequence, there has been an intense search for safer pesticides.

The all pervasive use of synthetics in every walk of life, be it agriculture, clothing, preservation or health-care is now paving way for a search for eco-friendly products. All communities, internationally, are today inclined to trust and rely more on green technology than ever before since the advent of modern science. The era of dependency on synthetic chemicals of the early and middle twentieth century prompted synthesis of newer chemicals as a panacea for all diseases and ailments. The conservative attitude of some societies, which depended on natural products in preference to the synthetic, was often credited to inertia or backwardness.

Happily, modern societies today, finding themselves confounded in the web of their creation are willing to revert to nature for remedies. It is in this that neem has staged a comeback and promises to hold centre stage in the coming years.

Pesticides made from neem are products of natural plant origin. They are biodegradable and non-toxic. Neem products produce no ill-effects to humans and animals; they have no residual effect on agriculture produce. For these reasons neem is considered as the best substitute to hazardous pesticides.

With the current thrust on sustainable agriculture and organic farming, the use of botanical products as pesticides has acquired greater significance. Neem is a highly suitable candidate for environment-friendly, safe agriculture development. Azadirachtin can be used in agriculture and public health as an eco-friendly chemical. Use of neem products for plant protection will reduce the demand for chemical pesticides and thereby reduce the environmental load of these synthetic pesticides.

Synthetic pesticides are also a major source of health problems. With the use of bio-pesticides, farmers can avoid health hazards which frequently occur both in developed and developing countries.

Neem is extremely beneficial to save the environment from pollution; since its inflorescence is purifying 'with its feathery crests tossing fifty feet into the sky' neem is a veritable "Kalpataru" for giving healthy environs. Like other trees, it exhales out oxygen and keeps the oxygen level in the atmosphere balanced. Like other trees, it also brings other environmental benefits such as flood control, reduced soil erosion and less salination. Neem can avert environmental crisis in India and other tropical countries as it can be successfully used for rehabilitation of degraded ecosystems and wastelands. Neem is highly recommended for reforestation of semi-arid regions in India and tropics of the sub-Saharan region, Asia and Central America. Neem is extremely useful in urban forestry because it has remarkable ability to withstand air and water pollution as well as heat. Neem also helps in restoring and maintaining soil fertility which makes it highly suitable in agro-forestry.

Neem is a natural resource to keep environment clean. In villages and cities as well as on farms, it is useful as a windbreak. As a source of shade, it is excellent for parks, roadsides etc. Because of its so many qualities, it is a common practice in rural India to have a tree of neem within the compounds of most of the houses. Neem is also a regarded as a valuable forestry species in India.

ENVIRONMENTAL SERVICE RENDERED BY NEEM

Neem in Indian culture has been ranked higher than

'Kalpavriksha', the mythological wish-fulfilling tree. In 'Sharh-e-Mufridat Al-Qanoon', neem has been named as 'Shajar-e-Mubarak', 'the blessed tree', because of its highly beneficial properties. Although scientific studies are wanting, neem is reputed to purify air and the environment of noxious elements. Its shade not only cools but prevents the occurrence of many diseases.

During hot summer months in northern parts of the Indian subcontinent, the temperature under the neem tree is 10° C less than the surrounding temperature; 10 air conditioners operated together may not do the job as efficiently and economically as a full grown neem. Restoration of the health of degraded soils and ultimate use of such reclaimed wastelands lands through neem is another example of its value as an environmental panacea.

About a decade ago, some 50,000 neem trees were planted over 10 kms on the Plains of Arafat to provide shade for Muslim pilgrims during hajj. The neem plantation has had a marked impact on the area's microclimate, microflora, microfauna, sand soil properties, and when full grown could provide shade to 2 million pilgrims. It is an ancient belief that neem growing inside the house can keep the surrounding air clean of impurities and thereby control environmental pollution. Also, hanging neem twigs on the door of a house is said to offer protection against pollution and disease.

The tree is not only beautiful to look at, providing grandeur and serenity, but also serves as a refuge to many beneficial organisms, bats, birds, honey bees, spiders, etc. Honey-combs established on the neem tree are singularly free from the galleria wax moth infestation. Many species of birds and fruit-eating bats subsist on the sweet flesh of ripe fruits, while certain rodents selectively feed on the kernel, confirming neem's safety to warm-blooded animals. The litter of falling leaves improves soil fertility and the organic content. Presently, little is known about the mycorrhizal associations between neem and bacterial and fungal endophytes, but the tree seems to be a living microcosm.

The evergreen, perennial tree can survive up to from 200 to 300 years, if not cut down. Even a highly conservative estimate of the 'environmental service' rendered by the tree @ US $ 10 per month, would give an astonishing value of US $ 24,000 to 36,000 in its life time. Other economic uses of neem and the benefits derived, such as biomass production, timber, seed and honey are more tangible and quantifiable.

NEEM IN REFORESTATION AND AGRO-FORESTRY

Neem appears to be a good candidate for planting throughout most of the warmer parts of the world. It not only grows vigorously in many types of semiarid and tropical sites, it is a versatile species that provides villagers with various products from which to derive an income during the years when the trees are maturing. It is also promising for planting in areas now suffering desperate fuelwood shortages. This feature is important for motivating enthusiastic local tree planting.

This tree is a farmer's friend and, when people know it better, it is likely to stimulate much spontaneous planting, especially as markets for its fruits and seeds develop. On the farm and around the house neem is useful not only as a windbreak and a welcome source of shade, but its seedcake is a good fertilizer-containing nitrogen, potash, phosphorus, calcium, and magnesium.

Neem is a very valuable forestry species in India and Africa and is also becoming popular in Tropical America, the middle-east countries and in Australia. Being a hardy, multipurpose tree, it is ideal for reforestation programs and for rehabilitating degraded, semiarid and arid lands. During a severe drought in Tamil Nadu State in June-July 1987, it was witnessed that neem grew luxuriantly, while other vegetation dried up.

Neem is useful as windbreaks and in areas of low rainfall and high wind speed. In the Majjia Valley in Niger, over 500 km of windbreaks comprised of double rows of neem trees have been planted to protect millet crops which resulted in a 20% increase in grain yield. Neem, windbreaks on a smaller scale have also been grown along sisal plantations in coastal Kenya. Large scale planting of neem has been initiated in the Kwimba Afforestation Scheme in Tanzania.

In countries from Somalia to Mauritiania, neem has been used for halting the spread of the Sahara desert. Also, neem is a preferred tree along avenues, in markets, and near homesteads because of the shade it provides. However, neem is best planted in mixed stands. It was probably no coincidence that Emperor Ashoka, the great ruler of ancient India, in the 3rd century BC, commanded that the neem be planted along the royal highway and roads along with other perennials-tamarind, *Tamarindus indica* and mahua, *Madhuca longifolia* var. *latifolia*. Neem has all the good characters for various social forestry programs.

Neem is an excellent tree for silvipastoral system involving production of forage grasses and legumes. But according to some reports, neem cannot be grown among agricultural crops due to its aggressive habit. Others say that neem can be planted in combination with fruit cultures and crops such as sesame, cotton, hemp, peanuts, beans, sorghum, cassava, etc., particularly when neem trees are still young. The neem tree can be lopped to reduce shading and to provide fodder and mulch. Recent advances in tissue culture and biotechnology should make it possible to select neem phenotypes with desirable height and stature for use in intercropping and various agro-forestry systems. The allelopathic effects of neem on crops, if any, need to be investigated.

BIOMASS PRODUCTION AND UTILIZATION

Full grown neem trees yield between 10 to 100 tons of dried biomass/ha, depending on rainfall, site characteristics, spacing, ecotype or genotype. Leaves comprise about 50% of the biomass; fruits and wood constitute one-quarter each. Improved management of neem stands can yield harvests of about 12.5 cubic meter (40 tons) of high quality solid wood/ha.

Neem wood is hard and relatively heavy and religious icons in some parts of India. The wood seasons well, except for end splitting. Being durable and termite resistant, neem wood is used in making fence posts, poles for house construction, furniture etc. There is growing market in some European countries for light-colored neem wood for making household furniture. Pole wood is especially important in developing countries; the tree's ability to resprout after cutting and to regrow its canopy after pollarding makes it highly suited to pole production. Neem grows fast and is a good source of firewood and fuels; the charcoal has high calorific value.

Chapter **20**

Sustainable Development and Environmental Conservation

The population in India has already crossed the one billion marks. Providing adequate food entitlements, safeguarding public health, meeting fuel and firewood needs, and at the same time preventing deforestation and conserving the environment, and slowing down the population growth will be daunting challenges in the coming decades. Although "green revolution technologies" have more than doubled the yield potential of cereals, especially rice and wheat in India, these high-input production systems requiring large quantities of fertilisers, pesticides, irrigation, and machines disregard the ecological integrity of land, forests, and water resources, endanger the flora and fauna, and cannot be sustained over generations. Future food security and economic development would depend on improving the productivity of biophysical resources through the application of sustainable production methods, by improving tolerance of crops to adverse environmental conditions, and by reducing crop and post-harvest losses caused by pests and diseases. Appropriate technologies, which do not assault the nature, would have key roles to play in ensuring food security, in improving public and animal health, and in rehabilitating the environment to safeguard the wellbeing of the posterity. Instead of striving for more "green revolutions" with emphasis on miracle seeds, hard-hitting synthetic and engineered pesticides, and increased use of fertilisers, the future must look to natural ways and processes for augmenting agricultural productivity. In fact, all development efforts and activities, including pest management, should be within well-defined ecological rules rather than within narrow economic gains. Sustainable agricultural systems must be efficient (i.e. effective and economically rewarding) and ecologically sound for long-term food sufficiency, equitable in providing social justice, ethical in respecting both future generations and other species, and lead to employment- and income-generating opportunities. For India, the use of neem may provide a key component in more sustainable agricultural systems, including pest and nutrient management, animal health, human health, and environmental conservation.

According to a report of an ad hoc panel of the Board on Science and Technology for International Development, "this plant(neem) may usher in a new era in pest control, provide millions with inexpensive medicines, cut down the rate of human population growth and even reduce erosion, deforestation, and the excessive temperature of an overheated globe." Neem's other descriptions, such as "nature's bitter boon," "nature's gift to mankind," "the tree for many an occasion," "the tree that purifies," "the wonder tree," "the tree of the 21st century," and "a tree for solving global problems," are a recognition of its versatility. Its botanic name, Azadirachta indica, derived from Farsi, "azad darakht-i-hindi" literally means the "free or noble tree of India," suggesting that it is intrinsically free from pest and disease problems and is benign to the environment. Neem's Sanskrritized name "Arishtha" means the reliever of sickness. In East African Kiswahili language, neem is known as "Mwarubaini," meaning the reliever of 40 disorders.

A full-grown tree can produce 30- to 100kg of fruits, depending on rainfall, insolation, soil type, and ecotype or genotype. Fifty kg of fruit yields 30kg of seed, which gives 6kg of oil and 24kg of seed cake. Neem has more than 100 unique bioactive compounds, which have potential applications in agriculture, animal care, public health, and for even regulating human fertility.

Neem has had a long history of use primarily against household and storage pests and to some extent against crop pests in India. With the advent of broad-spectrum, toxic insecticides, such as DDT, the use of neem in crop protection declined. However, over the past three decades, neem has come under close scientific scrutiny as a source of unique natural products for integrated pest management, medicine, industry, and other purposes. In spite of high selectivity, neem derivatives affect 500 species of insect pests belonging to different insect orders, one species of ostracods, several species of mites and ticks, nematodes, and even noxious snails and fungi, and aflatoxin-producing *Aspergillus* spp.

Results of large-scale field trials conducted by me and others in major food crops, such as rice, maize, sorghum, banana, and vegetables, such as kale, cabbage, cauliflower, cucumber, okra, tomato, potato, etc., have illustrated the value of neem-based pest management for enhancing crop productivity. The use of neem and fertiliser mixtures can reduce ammonia volatilisation loss caused by nitrifying bacteria in soil, thus effecting saving on fertilisers. A large number of neem-based medicines, pharmaceuticals, and toiletries are being produced today and are in great demand overseas. Neem oil is in great demand for treating skin infections, foot rot, ringworm, scabies, lice, burn wounds, bruises, etc. in humans and against ticks, mites, and blood-sucking flies in livestock. Neem has scope in reforestation and agro-forestry ad rehabilitating waste- and degraded lands. It is useful as windbreaks and in areas of low rainfall and high wind speed, it can protect crops from desiccation. In some countries in Africa, neem is being used for halting the spread of the Sahara desert. A full-grown neem tree does the job of 10 air conditioners; the temperature under the neem tree is 10 oC less than the outside ambient temperature. The ecological and economic service rendered by a neem tree in its lifetime of 250 years approximates US$24,000. In India, 6 million neem trees can easily be planted along the east-west and north-south corridors. Rural population along those corridors can be trained and employed to do the job scientifically. Once full grown, these trees will help in sequestering carbon emission and also reduce the load of greenhouse gases. The economic and ecological returns from such a programme will be phenomenal and India would become a role model for other tropical countries.

The neem industry has been growing steadily. Although presently India has 22 million neem trees (the largest concentration of neem in the world), the situation may change drastically. Neem trees of superior ecotypes and genotypes are being planted on a large scale in China and Brazil, countries much bigger than India in land area. Over the past 5 years, 20 million neem trees have been grown in Yunnan and other southern provinces of China. Neem also is being grown in some regions in Australia, in many countries in Africa, Latin America, Caribbean Islands, etc. For instance, 600,000 neem trees have been planted on homesteads and in plantations in Kwimba Reforestation Project in Mwanza, Tanzania. Likewise, in refugee rehabilitation centres near the river Nile at Adjumani, northern Uganda, about 200,000 neem trees were grown in pure stands and mixed plantations. Under this scenario, if no action is taken to promote neem in India, then we will be left far behind in the production of raw neem material and value-added neem products.

Neem has much to offer in solving agricultural and public health problems in the country, especially in rural areas. However, more neem trees will have to be grown to meet the increasing demand for insect pest control and industrial uses. The local peasant community will have to be brought within the fold of increased awareness by outreaching and through interpersonal interaction, by involving 'sarpanch' or village chiefs, schools, women groups, and government and non-government organisations. Field demonstrations and neem fairs at strategic locations will have to be organised periodically in collaboration with local bodies or institutions to evoke the interest and participation of target communities. Also, existing local initiatives, if any, will have to be strengthened.

Strategies for creating awareness will involve hands-on training through lectures and demonstrations to trainers, comprising agricultural trainers, foresters, extension personnel, health workers, teachers, journalists, and representatives of NGOs, youth and women groups, who would then have a multiplier effect in target areas. They will have to be taught how to harvest, collect and process neem seed, grow and plant seedlings, and use various neem materials for pest management. The distribution of raw materials will have to be guaranteed by establishing nodal agencies in target areas. These activities will create employment opportunities and also generate income.

The complex molecular structure of bio-active neem compounds precludes their chemical synthesis economically. Therefore, even the chemical industry will have to rely on the use of raw material. With growing demand for natural pest control materials, the use of neem products is becoming popular worldwide. In the next 5 years, I expect that global neem trade, comprising neem-based pest control materials, medicines, pharmaceuticals, and toiletries will grow to more than $500m. Herein lies a huge window of opportunity to benefit by growing and harnessing neem not only for local use but also for export to regions and countries where neem does not thrive.

Chapter **21**

Greening India with Neem

The human population of India=100 crore and growing @1 neem tree per 10 Indians, the needed numbers of neem tree = 10 crore minimum.

The current number of neem trees growing in India = 2 crore.

WHAT IS THE 'GREENING INDIA WITH NEEM' CAMPAIGN ALL ABOUT?

Greening India with neem is about giving people a choice to act. It is a growing movement in more ways than one! All around us there is talk that our planet is in crisis...... that we are destroying and polluting our way to a global catastrophe. We are repeatedly reminded that we have lost respect for the earth in our greed for speed, comfort and commercial gain.........

'Greening India with Neem' is a programme initiated by the Neem Foundation to channelize the growing concern of Indians about the environment into positive action. Keeping in view that deforestation, increasing soil salinity, accelerating soil erosion, over - grazing, automobile pollution and noxious emissions from industry are problems which affect a large majority of Indians, this programme aims to mobilize large scale public and government participation.

Each one of us is aware and worried about the ozone hole, the atmospheric warming, deforestation and the dire consequences of not taking action to address these problems.............. yet we all watch helplessly as cars, power stations and factories give out huge amounts of carbon dioxide and nitrogen oxides into the atmosphere and the earth becomes warmer. The concentration of CO_2 in the air has triggered climate change.

There is a real danger that global warming will lead to increases in the sea level. Besides warming is also beginning to affect rainfall patterns and food production.

The most effective action that an individual or a Greening Organization can take is to plant more neem trees. As this would lead to a healing chain reaction superior to any other! Trees absorb carbon dioxide and help maintain the delicate balance of oxygen and carbon dioxide in the atmosphere. Neem trees act as very efficient, natural air filters trapping dust particles, absorbing gaseous pollutants. The planting of neem trees helps reduce green house gases through photosynthesis absorbing large quantities of CO_2 and producing oxygen. Besides neem has remarkable ability to withstand air and water pollution, as well as heat. Neem also restores and maintains soil fertility.

WHY NEEM?

Neem is ecologically very special. It can tolerate very high levels of pollution and has the capacity to recover even if most of its foliage is dropped. Plants with a large leaf area such as neem, accumulate relatively higher quantities of lead. Trees vary widely in their capacity to absorb pollutants like particulate dust, CO_2 , oxides of sulphur and nitrogen. A study of locations in New Delhi, done by National Environmental Engineering Research Institute, India in 1996 indicated that neem tree is one of the most suitable species for checking urban pollution in industrial locations and it has potential in green belt development in hot spots with known history of high air pollution.

It was no coincidence that Emperor Ashoka, in the 3rd century before Christ, commanded that neem be planted along the road highway and roads along with other perennials, *Tamarindus indica* and *Madhuca latifolia*.

Neem has relatively high efficiency of CO_2 fixation. It can fix more than 14 umole of CO_2 per m^2 Sec. With a thick foliage canopy and a very high leaf surface area, it provides a good option for maximum CO_2 fixation and providing a shield against other pollution components particularly SO_2.

WHEN DID IT BEGIN?

The Neem Foundation first began its efforts to enthuse Indians about the neem tree in 1993. By 1997 it realized that many, many more neem trees would be needed if all the potential uses of this extremely versatile tree were to be tapped. Also realized that it would take a minimum of ten years for the trees to mature, so even if began planting them without delay, it would still take a decade.

Keeping this in mind the Foundation approached the Ministry of Environment and Forests in Delhi with a request that while according environmental / forest clearance a stipulation/ condition should be made that '*Azadirachta indica* should be planted as one of the species in the Afforestation / Green belt development programme'.

In January 1998, the Neem Foundation decided to take up the challenge and set a national target based on the demographic realities. Thus the idea of **'Greening India with Neem'** took shape.

In September 1998 in order to ensure that the neem tree receives priority in the Govt. of India, afforestation and eco-development programmes the Foundation invited the Hon. Minister for Environment and Forests Shri Suresh Prabhu to interact with its members and experts. As a result of this interaction the ministry convened a two day zonal conference following which it was decided to incorporate neem in Forestry and Social Forestry Programmes on a national scale.

As neem has a vital role to play in making agriculture sustainable the Ministry of Agriculture, Govt. of India through the NOVOD Board invited the Foundation, as one of two NGO's and nine premier Government Institutes to be part of the National Neem Network to implement a National Programme on neem. The Neem Foundation worked in close co-operation with the reputed Organizations from 1999 - 2002 to promote and facilitate neem plantation on a large scale by identifying, raising and providing superior neem germplasm.

The 3-year programme was successfully undertaken by the Foundation. 30,00,000 neem saplings from superior genotypes were raised and distributed under this programme.

Having created a space for the neem tree in the modern Indian psyche, the Neem Foundation approached the eminent film personality and Member of Parliament **Mrs. JAYA BACHCHAN**, for energizing the movement to carry the message of large scale plantation of neem through the media. On being appraised of the hurdles and challenges being faced by the neem movement, she willingly agreed and a TV and radio campaign featuring her has been launched.

WHY IS THE TARGET 10 CRORE NEEM TREES?

By rough estimates, India **currently has about 2 crore (20 million) neem trees. The population of India is almost 100 crore (1 billion)**. The equation works out to approx. 1 neem tree for every 50 Indians. This proportion is grossly inadequate, keeping in view that every part of this fascinating plant is packed with anti-bacterial, anti-fungal, anti-viral, anti-histamine, anti-septic and immune stimulating compounds for treating hundreds of maladies.

Neem has a long record of safety to human health and wide acceptability as a herbal medicine. It is one of the few trees that has withstood modern scientific scrutiny. Neem boosts the immune system on all levels while helping the body fight infection even before the immune system is called into action. Unlike synthetic antibiotics, neem does not destroy beneficial bacteria and other micro organisms needed to maintain optimum health. Neem offers a non-toxic alternative to powerful and sometimes damaging prescription medicines. It also has powerful skin rejuvenating qualities. Therefore increasing the number of neem trees to about 1 for every 10 Indians would have great impact in improving public health, especially in the rural areas where health care facilities are minimal.

The other major factor that influenced the final target was that India has today more than 100 million hectares of barren, unproductive and degraded wastelands. Even a token target of planting 1 neem tree per hectare of wasteland could help drive home the message of using our own biological heritage and knowledge to make productive use of our nation's natural resources.

WHO CAN JOIN HANDS?

Each and every person concerned about the degradation of the environment and the threat to future generations, whether in India or elsewhere is welcome to join the movement. **'Greening India with Neem'** is very much a people's initiative and will remain so.

It is being implemented by bringing together on a single platform –

- Individuals
- Village Communities
- Panchayats
- State Governments
- Government Bodies
- Non-Government Organizations
- Semi-Government Organizations
- Schools
- Hospitals
- Agricultural Universities
- Corporations
- Trusts
- Institutions
- NRIs
- PIO
- Funding Bodies

HOW MANY NEEM TREES SHOULD ONE PLANT?

While there is no limit to the number of neem trees that one can plant, the limitation is normally the availability of land and suitable sites. In case you are unable to find a suitable site to plant your own neem, you can still help by talking about this cause to as many people as possible. If each one of us can inspire a few others to plant neem trees, the job will be done and nature will take care of rest.

WHERE CAN WE PLANT THE TREES?

Neem trees can be planted in:

- Housing Societies – to repel mosquitoes and to enhance the availability of oxygen.
- Road sides - to provide cooling shade and to reduce CO_2, SO_2 levels.
- Parks – to provide a CO_2 sink, to purify the air and provide refuge for birds.
- Highways - to absorb the pollutants and provide shade.
- Around farm lands – to act as wind breaks, to bind soil against erosion and to provide natural home grown pest control material.
- They can be planted practically any location that receives plenty of sunlight and does not get water logged during rains.

HOW WILL WE BENEFIT FROM THIS PROGRAMME AS A NATION?

Greening India with Neem is a long term environmental programme aimed at providing one neem tree for every 10 Indians, so that Indians can use it freely for health and hygiene as well as for organic agriculture and all other known uses.

The neem tree is globally being acknowledged as the most valuable tree in the world, in terms of commercial and industrial potential. The neem tree is the de-facto National Tree of India. It is the grand old tree of the Indian countryside and can make a cleaner, greener and more fertile India a reality!

Chapter 22

World Neem Conference

THE EVENT

NEEM 2006- World Neem Conference

11th - 13th October, Mauritius

It is with immense pleasure that we announce the 5th World Neem Conference to be held in the beautiful Island Republic of Mauritius.

The Event is being organized by the Neem Foundation in collaboration with University of Mauritius, which will also be the venue for the Conference. Several other important agencies of Mauritius like

- Faculty of Agriculture, University of Mauritius
- The Food & Agricultural Research Council
- Mauritius Sugar Industry Research Institute
- Ministry of Environment, Govt. of Mauritius
- Agriculture Research & Extension Unit

have pledged their co-operation and support.

The Conference will showcase the latest research efforts in neem from around the world. As the world has moved rapidly on since the last conference on neem which was in 2002, newer trends and dimensions to the potential of *Azadirachta indica* will be presented and discussed.

It will also provide an opportunity to understand and define the role of neem in meeting sustainability challenges. Given that the success of the UN Millennium Development Goals (MDGs) could dramatically alter the condition of the world's disadvantaged, the Conference will provide a platform for stake holders to evaluate technologies based on neem that have potential for uplifting and enhancing the quality of life, the world over.

UN Millennium Development Goals

1. Eradicate extreme poverty and hunger.
2. Achieve universal primary education.
3. Promote gender equality and empower women.
4. Reduce child mortality.
5. Improve maternal health.
6. Combat HIV / AIDS, malaria and other diseases.
7. Ensure environmental sustainability.
8. Develop a global partnership for development.

As this three day Event will also aim to promote the sharing of experiences from countries and agencies that have implemented or are embarking on their own neem programmes, we hope you will make the most of this rare opportunity.

Come to Mauritius to join this gathering to personally interact with Neem Experts, Scientists, Researchers, Scholars, Developmental Organizations, Administrators, Organic Growers, Processors and Industrialists.

THE THEME

'NEEM: GREEN TECHNOLOGY FOR A SAFER WORLD'

THEME AREAS OF NEEM 2006

- Chemistry
- Genetic Improvement & Afforestation
- Insect Control
- Nematode Control
- Fungus Control
- Fertilizer Use Efficiency
- Environmental Issues
- Socio-Economic Issues
- Human Health

- Animal Health
- Ecological Aspects of Neem
- Neem for the entrepreneur
- Registration & Regulatory Implications
- Processing & Product Development
- Neem Product Registration
- Neem in Bio-technology
- Organized Neem Plantations
- Legal Processes
- Global Perspective
- Others

GENESIS

The Neem Tree - *Azadirachta indica* with its versatile use-profile is increasingly being recognised as the most valuable tree on Earth. During the First International Neem Conference 1980, held at Rottachegrern, Germany, it was noted that many scientists all over the world have studied neem components, but these efforts have been both isolated and sporadic. It was suggested that measures should be taken on a national, regional and international basis to co-ordinate and promote results in a practical context.

The Second International Neem Conference was held in 1983 at Rauischholzhausen, in Germany. Three years later, the Third International Neem Conference was held in Nairobi.

Subsequently, the first World Neem Conference was held in Bangalore, India in February 1993. It was the largest gathering so far on the subject. More than 400 delegates from 30 countries participated. It was a showcase of tremendous worldwide efforts related to the various aspects and possibilities of neem. The flow of information and exchange of ideas about the research and studies of dedicated people throughout the world was phenomenal.

The Second World Neem Conference was held at Gatton College near Brisbane, Australia in February 1996. Over a 100 delegates from 20 countries participated.

The third World Neem Conference was held in May 1999, at the University of British Columbia, Vancouver, Canada under the aegis of the Neem Foundation. There were about 120 delegates from 24 countries. 58 papers and 23 posters were presented. An analysis of the paper and poster presentation in Vancouver reveals interesting and encouraging facts about the inspiration that the Neem Tree provides. This phenomenon cuts across borders and promotes international co-operation.

During the course of the Conference, the delegates widely appreciated the genesis and outcome of the Conference and it was unanimously decided to hold the next World Neem Conference in India in 2002.This suggestion was accepted and Neem Foundation, being the apex body for all neem movements globally, took the lead in organizing the Fourth World Neem Conference in Mumbai. Prestigious national and international Scientific Bodies, Academies, Research Organizations, Funding Agencies, Industry and Government Departments are being invited to co-sponsor this prestigious International Conference and provide support and financial assistance.

Given the unprecedented global interest and research efforts in the neem tree today, Neem 2002 is widely anticipated to be the largest congregation of the neem fraternity ever.

Neem 2002, the 4th World Neem Conference was held in Mumbai from 27th - 30th November. The Conference was attended by all those who hold an interest in neem - from scientists, research scholars, policy makers, entrepreneurs and industrialists to organic growers.

During the four day deliberations about 140 papers were presented, divided into 18 sessions. There were in all 90 oral presentations divided into 16 sessions and 51 poster presentations divided into 2 sessions.

As the neem tree holds the promise of providing entrepreneurial opportunities and employment at the village level in Asia and Africa.

CALL FOR PAPERS

All those interested in neem and related fields are invited to submit an Abstract of a Paper for scrutiny at the Secretariat of the World Neem Conference.

Guidelines

- Abstract must be presented in English and must not be more than 300 words.
- The full names of all authors contributing to the paper and their institutional affiliations must be mentioned.
- The email / postal address should be included.
- Please mention clearly whether it is for oral or poster presentation.
- The abstract should be sent as a separate file and transmitted as an attachment in case it is being submitted via email.
- In case it is submitted on a floppy / CD, the author, abstract title should be written on the label.
- The software preferred would be MS-Word ('95 or latest version).
- Kindly refer to the important deadlines mentioned below for last date of submission.

Important Deadlines

Submission of Abstracts	-	28th February 2006
Acceptance of Papers	-	31st March 2006
Receipt of full length Papers	-	30th June, 2006

Chapter 23

Patent

The neem tree originates from the Indian subcontinent and now grows in the dry regions of more than 50 tropical countries around the world. The neem tree has multiple uses. It is mentioned in Indian texts written over 2000 years ago and has been used for centuries by local communities in agriculture as an insect and pest repellent, in human and veterinary medicine, toiletries and cosmetics. It is also venerated in the culture, religions and literature of the region.

Even though first report on pesticide property of neem was reported in India in 1928, only after 30 years later systematic research work on neem was initiated. The past five decades witnessed intensive investigation and upward trend to scientific interest in neem and its diverse properties, resulting in large number of research publications, books and conferences at national and international levels. It led to isolation and identification of hundreds of the active compounds, from various parts with pesticidal, nematicidal, fungicidal, bactericidal, anti inflammatory, anti-tumor and other properties and found its applications in pesticide, medical, healthcare and cosmetic industry all over the world.

Since the 1980s, many neem related process and products have been patented in Japan, USA and European countries. The first US patent was obtained by Terumo Corporation in 1983 for its therapeutic preparation from neem bark. In 1985 Robert Larson from (USDA) obtained a patent for his preparation of neem seed extract and the Environmental Protection Agency approved this product for use in US market. In 1988 Robert Larson sold the patent on an extraction process to the US Company W.R. Grace (presently Certis). Having gathered their patents and clearance from the EPA, four years later, Grace commercialized its product by setting up manufacturing plant in collaboration with P.J. Margo Pvt. Ltd. in India and continued to file patents from their own research in USA and other parts of world. Aside from Grace, neem based pesticides were also marketed by another company, AgriDyne Technologies Inc., USA, the market competition between the two companies was intense. In 1994, Grace accused AgriDyne a non-exclusive royalty-bearing license. During this period in India large number of companies also developed stabilized neem products and made them available commercially. The number of patents filed in this period were limited and geographically confined to few countries.

The challenge to a neem based patent held by W.R. Grace & Co. has returned many of intellectual property related issues controversies to center-stage globally. These two cases not only created a global awareness on neem and its properties but also raised issues on biopiracy, need for documentation of traditional knowledge, equitable sharing of gains from traditional knowledge and harmonization of patent rule. Success of revocation of European patent illustrates the requirement of systematic documentation of knowledge whether traditional or scientific. Further these cases demonstrate the potential of IPR in creating awareness, enthusiasm in scientists, entrepreneurs, organizations and society and increased investments in research and development of products which compete in the market place. This is evident from upward trend of patents filed globally on neem from 1994 - 96 onwards - intense patent debate period and commercial product available in markets from neem.

Largest number of patents is in USA (54) followed by Japan (35), Australia (23), India (14). In India additionally more than 53 patent applications are pending for either gazette notification or opposition since 1995. If granted India will have the largest number of patents in neem. This itself illustrates that IPR does not stifle creativity and innovation but creates challenges and opportunities to overcome the existing patents barriers by innovation and invention. There is also an increasing trend of filing application through PCT.

An analysis of type of patents suggests that majority of them are for crop protection applications (63%), followed by health care (13%), industrial (5%), veterinary care (5%), cosmetics (6%) and others (8%). This trend is also shown in country wise granted patents. For example in US out of 54 patents granted 31 were for crop protection rest for healthcare, cosmetics, industrial and veterinary applications. Organization wise patents ownership indicates largest number owned by Certis - W.R. Grace (49) followed by Rohm & Haas (36), CSIR-India (14), Trifolio (9), Bayer (8) and EID Parry (6).

The neem tree has been recognized the world over as a commercial opportunity. This is a welcome sign - but the bio-diversity prospects of this tree cannot be a free access to the entire world. It is now utterly urgent that the genetic fingerprints of our traditional wealth like neem are properly documented. It has repeatedly pointed out that an immensely potential plant like neem should not be just left unrecognized and unprotected.

Granting neem the status of National Tree would send out the right signals to the world. This one move will help convert a national resource into a national asset.

The Tea Tree of Australia, Gingko Biloba of China, Ginseng of Korea, Guarana of the Amazon and Aloe Vera of Mexico are huge money-spinners in the booming alternate therapy market place of the West. Neem of India can emerge as the biggest player of them all - if India wakes up in time, takes charge and leads by farming policies and encouraging its use in its farmlands and public health programs.

A small country like Korea could successfully globalize its national treasure GINSENG - with an integrated approach, active research and development and positive promotion. It is a hallmark of the success of Korean farmers and Governmental efforts. India must draw lessons from this example.

In early 90s, the European Patent Office granted patents to the US Department of Agriculture and Multinational Agricultural

Corporation (W.R. Grace of USA)

The patent was rejected on the basis that products derived from genetic resources (like peanut oil, sugarcane, corn, etc.) cannot be patented. There were about 50 companies that tried to get patents on Neem Products and about 70 patents were rejected. This dropped interest of Neem Oil by multinational mega corporation in agricultural area.

Chapter 24

Is Neem Safe?

How Neem Works on the Biochemical Level

Because neem is new to Western scientists, the number of pharmacological studies on neem has been somewhat limited. In those studies that have been made, the general conclusion is that neem not only kills some infective organisms directly but also boosts the immune response on several levels. This increases the body's ability to fight bacterial, viral, and fungicidal infections itself.

This combination of effects is more effective in the long run because chemicals toxic enough to eliminate all microbes often also harm healthy body tissue and cause undesirable side-effects. An improved immune system can selectively wipe out the invading microbes without adversely affecting other cells.

When invaded by microbes (or anything else the body recognizes as foreign), the immune system releases antibodies that lock onto and neutralize the intruder.

Neem not only enhances antibody production but also seems to improve the cell-mediated immune response by which white blood cells are unleashed to kill the invaders.

In this type of immune response, special scavenger cells in the blood called macrophages devour the microbes and present bits of them along with their own surface molecules. It is only after macrophages (or other antigen-presenting cells) present bits of the microbe as antigens that helper T cells recognize the antigens. These helper T cells then release chemical messengers called cytokines that galvanize other cells of the immune system into a counter-attack.

By enhancing the body's first line of defence, neem helps the immune system more quickly respond to infections that might otherwise gain a strong foothold that would then be more difficult to overcome.

Major Active Constituents of Neem

Figuring out exactly how a herb works and which compound or combinations of compounds are making it work is difficult. Constituting possibly hundreds of compounds, some active and others not, herbs are usually analyzed for their most active compound. This is done by systematically isolating each compound and determining its structure. This can show the class of chemical it belongs to and can indicate what type of effect it can be expected to have. With complex molecules, this process is very time-consuming, very expensive and often frustrating.

Neem trees have many unique compounds that have been identified and others that are as yet unidentified. The more common and therefore the most analyzed compounds are as follows:

- **nimbin** - anti-inflammatory, anti-pyretic, antihistamine, anti-fungal
- **nimbidin** - anti-bacterial, anti-ulcer, analgesic, anti-arrhythmic, anti-fungal
- **nimbidol** - anti-tubercular, anti-protozoan, anti-pyretic
- **gedunin** - vasodilator, anti-malaria, anti-fungal
- **sodium nimbinate** - diuretic, spermicide, anti-arthritic
- **queceretin** - anti-protozoal
- **salannin** - repellent
- **azadirachtin** - repellent, anti-feedant, anti-hormonal

TOXICOLOGICAL PERSPECTIVE

Numerous studies of possible toxicity resulted in a determination that leaf and bark are very low in toxicity, especially when taken orally. But large doses of neem leaves taken internally have caused some side effects in some of the animals in which it was tested.

Extensive research has been conducted on neem oil extracts for regulatory agencies in several countries, including the United States, and has been found to be safe in limited dosage for short periods of time.

Tests on animals required by the Environmental Protection Agency that alcohol extracts of the seed produced no external irritation in rabbits and no toxic effects on mice when taken internally, even in very large amounts.

Some people taking neem oil internally experienced nausea and general discomfort which is the case with many of the compound containing oils.

Excessive consumption of raw neem oil has been implicated in reduced liver functioning.

The toxic effects of neem oil consumption has been disputed by some researchers that believe contamination with aflatoxin or inadvertent additions of the oil of the chinaberry tree, a related species to neem which known to be toxic, is the cause of the observed side effects observed.

CAUTIONARY STATEMENT

Neem is generally considered an extremely safe product, even after centuries of daily ingestion in India, where it is used as a toothbrush and placed with food to protect against insects, no danger has been documented.

Children in India and Africa eat neem fruit with great enjoyment during its fruiting season. Rats treated with neem oil in laboratory studies actually gained weight instead of showing ill effects.

A German study using oil from clean neem seeds showed no toxicity at doses in excess of 5,000 mg per kg.

Tests undertaken for the U.S. Environmental Protection Agency before the approval of a commercial neem product, Margosan-O, showed no or limited toxicity to rats, ducks, rabbits and bees.

Neem's safe use for thousands of years throughout south Asia may be a result of following the prescribed dosages prescribed by the medical practitioners they visited.

While consuming large amounts of neem is traditional in Asian and African cultures, caution is still recommended until further research is complete.

A WORD OF CAUTION

Medicines from plants should, of course, be treated with the same caution as medicines from laboratories. Neem oil seems to be of particular concern. Consuming it, although widely practiced in parts of Asia, is not recommended. Doses as small as 5 ml have killed infants, and animal studies showed acute toxicity at doses as low as 14-24 ml per kg of body weight. It seems possible that this was caused by contaminants rather than by the oil itself. In Germany, toxicological tests using oil obtained from clean neem kernels resulted in no toxicity, even at a concentration of 5,000 mg per kg of body weight in rats. Nonetheless, caution is called for.

The leaves or leaf extracts also should not be consumed by people or fed to animals over a long period. There are anecdotal reports of renal failure in Ghanaians who were drinking leaf teas as a malaria treatment

None of this should be confused with earlier statements. The compounds and seed-kernel extracts responsible for the insecticidal activity appear to be essentially nontoxic to mammals.

Chapter 25

The Reality

Although the possibilities seem almost endless, nothing about neem is yet definite. The scientists who are most enthusiastic over the plant and its potential admit that at this stage the evidence to support their expectations is tentative. Even within the world of pest control its eventual place is by no means clear.

The truth is that despite all its properties and promise, some impediments must be overcome and many uncertainties clarified before neem's potential can be fully realized. These obstacles are summarized in this chapter; more detail can be found in later chapters.

DISADVANTAGES

By and large, the limitations known today all seem surmountable. Indeed, they present exciting challenges to the scientific and economic development communities. Solving them may well bring a major new resource and a means for benefiting much of the world.

The greatest impediment to neem's commercial development may simply be a general lack of credibility, or even awareness, of what it is and what it can do. Neither the public, the majority of pesticide manufacturers, nor the health-care community in industrial countries now appreciate the plant or its promise. This is due in part to a lack of experience, in part to a lack of industrial interest (caused notably by the difficulty of patenting natural products), and in part to a lack of laboratory data to substantiate the claims. One researcher has called the neem scene an "uncharted jungle" of miscellaneous assertions, disconnected details, and limitless possibilities.

Genetic Variability

Another difficulty is caused by the fact that many of the neem trees scattered around the world are (for all intents and purposes) genetically distinct. This means that conclusions drawn from one may not be exactly applicable to the others. Extracts from neighboring trees, for instance, may differ in their mixtures of ingredients.

There is no current evidence that this has caused any practical problems. Eventually, however, certain elite types will undoubtedly be selected and propagated.

Lack of Registration

In an era when many people are desperately seeking alternatives to synthetic pesticides, it is ironic that neem's very uniqueness is slowing its acceptance by regulatory authorities. Neem components incapacitate pests by repelling them, stopping them from feeding, or upsetting their growth—only indirectly by killing them. Its varying modes of action, its complex and synergistic mixture of ingredients, and its lack of standardization all raise barriers that trouble pesticide regulators.

Lack of Standards

Writing regulations to cover neem has been made even more difficult because no standard of potency has yet been developed. For consistency of composition, a mixed product from nature cannot compete with a single molecule from a laboratory. For instance, the mix of active ingredients may vary with the sample's age, the locality where it was grown, the genes of the tree it came from, or the method by which the sample was handled or shipped. Moreover, the analytical techniques are tricky and, for the moment at least, the various reports of neem's level of efficacy cannot all be trusted.

Although the tree is easy to grow, the specific horticultural and climatic conditions that maximize its potency are still unknown. Extracts from trees grown in different parts of the world currently show differing levels of activity, and the relative differences vary with the types of insects being tested. Sorting out just how genetics and environment-not to mention handling methods and insect species influence neem's various ingredients is a knotty problem. Experience may eventually prove, for example, that the best-looking seeds from the fastest-growing trees on the most advantageous sites produce the poorest pesticides.

Conflicting Approaches

It is one of neem's strengths that its ingredients can be used in formulations from the crudest to the most sophisticated. On the one hand, in a remote Third World village farmers may take a sack of crushed neem kernels, dunk it (like a tea bag) in a barrel of water overnight, and use the resulting "neem tea" on their vegetable crops the next day. On the other hand, the isolation of individual neem ingredients is already being conducted in sophisticated factory settings in the United States. This produces highly purified and certifiably uniform products that are a world away from neem tea in a tub in Thailand.

Both approaches are valid, of course, but their needs, priorities, costs, and objectives are so vastly different that people working at the two extremes may appear (even to themselves) to be working at cross-purposes. To the uninitiated, the conflicting views can make the whole neem concept seem unreliable.

Economic Uncertainties

The commercial production of any materials derived from the fruit of a tree is necessarily constrained by nature. There are limitations of seasonal supply, the long wait for the trees to mature, and the difficulty of facing the whims of nature. (For instance, in India neem fruits drop during the late monsoon, a time when frequent rains make them hard to dry.

On the other hand, in many tropical nations neem pesticides should prove to be much cheaper than synthetic pesticides, and they could be homegrown rather than imported. However, they will never be totally without cost. Gathering and processing neem products takes time and effort. Even people "growing their own" will probably have to take time off from farming, fuel gathering, or other vital activities to harvest their neem seed. Moreover, if pests arrive during a season when fresh seeds are unavailable, facilities for storing the seeds for future use will be needed.

Contributing notably to the expense (at least in new plantings) is the delay of several years before the first crop can be gathered. Not only must the growers carefully nurture the young tree during its first year or so, they will begin getting returns only after its fifth year under normal conditions.

There can be other economic uncertainties as well. As we have noted, for instance, it is not yet known how best to manage the tree to optimize its production of pesticidal ingredients. Nor is it yet known if and how the mix or quality of the pest-control compounds will change in any economically meaningful way with the location, the climate, or the tree's age.

Handling Difficulties

Although neem products (seeds, extracts, or seedcake) are safe and easy to handle and apply, they are bulky and some samples smell like a dreadful cross between garlic and peanut butter.

There is at this point no method for mechanizing the process of collecting, storing, or handling the seeds. Nor is it yet known how to carry out these operations so that the pesticidal ingredients retain their fullest potency.

Geographical Limitations

Neem trees cannot be grown just anywhere. They are sensitive to frost and can be produced only in the warmer parts of the world. There is also mounting evidence that under dry conditions their growth and yield can be erratic and their susceptibility to pests high.

Planting Difficulties

The seed's short viability is a problem in introducing neem to new locations. Fresh seeds germinate well, but within weeks germination rates begin dropping off. This poses logistical difficulties for any tree-planting endeavors outside the areas where the tree now grows.

Silviculture Difficulties

At this stage at least, neem seems primarily suited for individual or group plantings within household compounds and villages, along roadsides and canals, in marketplaces and parks, and around the edges of fields. However, its production in organized commercial plantations in the long term might prove to be its greatest value.

Usually there is little difficulty with livestock eating the seedlings or saplings, but humans filching the foliage for medicinals or toothbrushes can be a problem.

Instability

When exposed to sunlight, neem products degrade and lose their pest-control properties. Typically, the crude extracts remain active for only eight days when exposed to the sun's ultraviolet rays.

Under sophisticated conditions this limitation can be overcome. The neem formulation being sold in the United States, for instance, contains sunscreens. When sprayed on plants, it remains effective for 2-3 weeks, and it can be stored for at least 2 years with little or no loss of potency.

Neem materials are also sensitive to high temperatures and must be stored in shady places.

These inherent instabilities can be exacerbated when the extracts are made under uncontrolled conditions, such as in a Third World village. For example, the active compounds may be inactivated by acids, alkalis, or other contaminants of local water supplies. Other types of pesticides might well be similarly affected, but neem extracts are more likely to be prepared where water is impure.

Health Hazards

Although neem has shown every indication of being safe to mammals in normal use as a pesticide (see Appendix A), the possibility of future hazards should not be dismissed. Few toxicity tests on higher mammals such as dogs, pigs, primates, or people have yet been published. As a result, in the United States neem products are not yet authorized for use on food crops. Their persistence in residues on foods is also unknown.

A known health hazard may arise as a result of poor handling. The harvested fruits must be depulped quickly and the seeds dried under shade and stored under shelter from the sun and rain. This is because at moisture contents above 14 per cent, the fruits can carry the fungus Aspergillus Flavus, which under many conditions produces aflatoxins. These are among the most potent carcinogens known and, unfortunately, they can contaminate the seeds inside the fruits. Indeed, they are extracted and concentrated along with the pesticidal ingredients. This may eventually prove to be the greatest barrier to the wider use of the pesticides from this most promising tree. It is, however, a problem only in the more humid neem-growing areas. Elsewhere, the climate is usually too dry for fungi to infect the fruits.

Environmental Safety

The fact that neem extracts are natural products does not mean that they are benign. Indeed, there is evidence that they can affect certain aquatic life. Most studies with fish in laboratory tests have shown no deleterious effects, but in one trial both tadpoles and the mosquito-eating fish gambusia died when neem extracts were applied to the water. And neem seeds falling into fish ponds in Haiti killed tilapia fry. These experiences do not necessarily indicate an environmental hazard—only that caution and more toxicological studies are needed. It seems likely that neem oil, rather than the other seed-kernel ingredients, is causing the toxicity.

Although using neem will seldom harm beneficial insects, there are a few cases of negative effects. There is, for instance, a report of it affecting the larvae of hover flies. Also, there may be other subtle secondary effects. Bees and butterflies drinking nectar from neem dosed plants might, for example, pick up traces of neem components, leading to reduced reproduction. The same may be said for insects that feed on other insects. To date, however, no evidence for such deleterious effects has surfaced.

Slow Action

Compared to DDT and other synthetic pesticides, the wait for neem to act may seem endless. Insects treated with it die by delayed action. Although their destructive power drops fast as the neem materials take effect, they may continue living for 2 weeks. Eventually, however, the next generation fails to emerge and the population collapses.

Although the end result may be more devastating than that from DDT, people used to seeing rapid knockdown may be initially disappointed, or even discouraged. This lack of quick effect poses a challenge for promoting neem in pest-control markets where people have come to expect instantaneous results

Damage to Plants

It is one of neem's most exciting features that its compounds are systemic. However, they are not systemic in all plant species. Potato plants, for example, do not take up the main active ingredient, azadirachtin, whereas beans do. This introduces yet another uncertainty. Each plant species may have to be checked individually. Also, the acidity of the soil or the level of enzymatic activity in the plant may affect the length of time that neem compounds remain effective inside the plant tissues.

Moreover, it has been found in greenhouse and field trials that certain neem materials can damage plants. In cabbages, for example, only medium-sized heads were formed. In onions, the waxy coating on the leaves was destroyed. In tomatoes, the growth and yield were reduced.

Much of this "phytotoxicity" was apparently due to neem oil contaminating the samples. There were large differences between the damage caused by crude fractions and by refined products. It could be, therefore, that only highly purified extracts can be reliably used for systemic purposes. At normal levels, these have so far proved safe to even sensitive plants.

Method of Application

Although neem products can be applied using standard equipment (both sophisticated and primitive), they may have specific requirements if they are to be fully effective. For example, some pests must be treated at a certain time of day. Colorado potato beetle is one. If potato fields are sprayed when the sun is high, the extracts dry out and have little effect. On the other hand, if sprayed at dawn, they can be extremely effective.

A product like this, which affects certain subtle aspects of an insect's life, is restricted by factors having to do with the insect's habits, life stage, and metabolic processes. In many cases the users will have to be educated, or at least trained, before neem can be fully effective.

Protecting the Tree

Despite the fact that it is a source of pesticidal materials, the tree itself is attacked by certain pests. In 1986, for example, an outbreak of the oriental yellow scale was confirmed in West Africa (see next chapter). This insect, a native of India and the Far East, defoliates and sometimes kills the tree. Recent reports suggest that it has severely damaged neem trees over large areas of northern Cameroon, Chad, northeastern Nigeria, and eastern Niger. It seems likely that this outbreak resulted from the stresses of a decade or more of drought in the Sahel, which has left many neems weak and sickly. Nonetheless, further devastating pest outbreaks are certainly possible.

Medical Limitations

Whereas millions of Indians swear to the efficacy of neem treatments, the pharmacological effects have seldom been subjected to rigorous trials with controls. Thus, to officials in many other parts of the world, today's claims of medical efficacy are suspect. Indeed, a couple of recent studies suggest that it may be unsafe to eat neem products.

One study (already mentioned) dealt with the use of neem oil as a general cure-all for children. It strongly suggests that this is a most unwise practice, at least among the very young. When children under the age of four were given doses (5-30 ml) of neem oil, they came down with a disease similar to Reye's syndrome. This severe disorder involves swelling of the brain, liver, and other organs. Both Reye's syndrome and its neem-oil-induced mimic are poorly understood. Nonetheless, the message is clear: neem oil and neem extracts should not be used for internal medicinal purposes until more thoroughly tested.

There are also anecdotal accounts from West Africa of neem-leaf teas possibly causing kidney damage when taken over a long period.

In other studies, neem extracts were found to be toxic to guinea pigs and rabbits and leaves fed to goats and guinea pigs (50-200 mg per kg body weight) reduced their rate of growth .

The ultimate significance of these preliminary studies is unclear. The materials used may well have been contaminated-perhaps by fungal toxins. Other trials have found no toxicity problem. For instance, in a toxicological study in Germany, neem oil obtained from clean, fungus-free seed kernels showed no oral toxicity in rats. The dosage tested was 5,000 mg per kg body weight .

Certainly, no hazard has been observed when neem has been used in topical treatments (on skin complaints, for example) or in dental uses-which together make up by far the major medical applications. Nor is there any evidence that using the seed-kernel extracts as pesticides is hazardous to health.

Whether neem oil is safe for possible use as an intravaginal spermicide is also unclear. However, in this use there are perhaps even greater uncertainties. Contraception is a topic of such sensitivity-personal, political, scientific, and religious-that here, too, its future role is uncertain.

Its use as a spermatocide-the male contraceptive mentioned earlier-is so uncertain that it will likely take decades of research to develop even if no safety hazards are found along the way.

Synthetic Competition

The number and complexity of the compounds in neem extracts will always preclude the economic synthesis of the full mixture. On the other hand, individual compounds may prove suitable for synthesis. There is, therefore, the possibility that if neem opens up a new generation of pesticides, synthetic mimics may capture some of the more lucrative "top-end" markets.

Appendix

DATA REQUIREMENTS FOR REGISTRATION OF NEEM BASED PESTICIDES

A.	CHEMISTRY	
1.	Name of the Part of the Plant(s) to be used for extraction of the active ingredients / components.	R
2.	Outline of process of manufacture clearly identifying the chemicals as indicated in point(3) below.	R
3.	(a) Neem extract Contains "Azadirachtin" as one of the major active constituents. The concentration of Azadirachtin in the formulated neem extract should contain not less than 1500 ppm of Azadirachtin a.i.in "Kernel" based formulations and 300 ppm in "Neem oil" based formulations.. (b) When the insecticidal a.i. is other than Azadirachtin then the applicant has to indicate the name, quality and quantity of that particular a.i. (s).	R
4.	Chemical identity of the ingredient as stated at point (3) above.	R
5.	Physico-chemical properties.	R
6.	Specifications of ingredient as indicated at point (3) above.	R
7.	Method of analysis for Azadirachtin / other insecticidal a.i. other than Azadirachtin.	R
8.	Analytical test report	R
10.	Shelf-life claim / data.	R
B.	BIO-EFFICACY	
1.	Bio-effectiveness	R
2.	Phytotoxicity	R
3.	Compatibility with other chemicals	R
4.	Purpose of manufacture	R
5.	Direction concerning dosage	R
6.	Time of application	R
7.	Waiting period	R
8.	Application equipment	R
9.	Information regarding registration status in other countries, if any	R

C.	**TOXICITY : Data on parameters 1 to 3 are required for 9(3b) registration.**	
1.	Acute oral rat and mice	R
2.	Acute dermal	R
3.	Primary skin irritation, irritation to mucous membrane.	R
4.	Neuro-behavioural toxicity	R
5.	Reproductive toxicity.	R
6.	Careinogenicity	R
7.	Mutagenicity	R
8.	Effect on spray operators (Health records) : As per the protocol to be approved by the Registration Committee.	R
D.	**PACKAGING AND LABELLING**	
1.	Labels and Leaflets as per IR 1971 existing norms	R
2.	Type of packaging (container content compatibility data)	R
3.	Manner of Labelling (Container - content compatibility data)	R
4.	Specification for primary package	R
5.	Specification for secondary package	R
6.	Specification for transport package	R
7.	Manner of labelling	R
8.	Instructions for storage and use	R
9.	Information regarding disposal of used package	R
10.	Process of manufacturing / indicating material balance generation of wasted.	R
11.	Long Term Toxicity	R
i.	Neuro-behaviour toxicity	R
ii.	Mutagenicity	R
iii.	Careinogenecity	R
iv.	Effect on reproduction	R
v.	Health records of workers / spray operators as per the protocol to be approved by the Registration Committee	R
E.	**PACKAGING & LABELLING**	
1.	Labels and Leaflets	R
2.	Type of packing	R

3.	Manner of packing	R
4.	Content container compatibility data shall be generated in an independent reputed laboratory.	R
5.	Manner of labelling	R
6.	Specifications of packing	R
	i. Primary packing	R
	ii. Secondary packing	R
	iii. Transport packing	R
7.	Instructions for storage and use	R
8.	Disposal of empty containers	R

R- Required

NR- Not required.

Index